Breastfeeding
OUTLOOK

How to Pass the IBLCE Exam This Time:

Making the Sure-Footed Climb to Success After Failure

Marie Biancuzzo, *RN MS CCL IBCLC*

Gold Standard Publishing

Graphics and Layout: *Breastfeeding Outlook*
Cover Design: *Breastfeeding Outlook*

A Note to the Reader
The author and publisher have made every attempt to check content for accuracy. Because the health care sciences are continually advancing, our knowledge base continues to expand. Therefore, we recommend that the reader check product information for changes in dosages, contraindications, and other information about any medication or intervention.

Marie Biancuzzo and Breastfeeding Outlook are not affiliated with IBLCE.

The International Board of Lactation Consultant Examiners® (IBLCE®) owns certain names, trademarks, and logos, including IBLCE and the certification marks International Board Certified Lactation Consultant® and IBCLC® (the "Marks"). Use of these Marks in this publication does not state or imply IBLCE endorsement.

A Request to the Reader
We invite your comments and constructive suggestions. If you find an error, please notify us at *info@breastfeedingoutlook.com*.

The most recent version of this document may always be obtained at *breastfeedingoutlook.com*

Breastfeeding Outlook
PO Box 387
Herndon VA 20172-0387
breastfeedingoutlook.com

ISBN # 978-1-931048-56-9

10 9 8 7 6 5 4 3 2

Preface

In the spring of 2004, I launched *Marie Biancuzzo's Lactation Exam Review* in Detroit. In the wee hours of the morning, I was frantically finishing a slide presentation that I would be using later that day. Looking back on it, I wonder how I taught that group anything useful.

I had a very limited idea of the content that people needed to review before taking the IBLCE exam. Sure, I had looked at the Detailed Content Outline (Formerly called the "Blueprint.") But in truth, I wasn't too sure what kinds of questions would be in those categories. What little I remembered about a past IBLCE exam was vague at best. I hadn't taken the IBLCE exam in 10 years; I was preparing myself—as well as the class—to take the exam about two months later.

Luckily, the Detroit group was fairly smart (and very forgiving!) The 2-day review went well. Since then, I have offered the course in over twenty cities, and I've developed an online version. I've taught literally thousands of people; 25% of the currently-certified IBCLCs in the United States have come through one or more of my courses. Unquestionably, it was seeing the struggles of the people sitting in the chairs that enabled me to continually improve the course.

Early on, I recognized that some course participants were not "reviewing" material. Many had never been exposed to the material. And, the few who had previously been exposed were often unable to connect the conceptual dots, or they hadn't retained the information they had learned. Others were so anxious that they made silly mistakes on the 50-question mock exam given on Day 2 of the course; when I gave them the results of their mock exams, many beat themselves up for having picked the wrong answer, because they knew better.

Later, I began to face another problem: People were coming to the review course because they had already failed the IBLCE exam. I tried to emphasize that this was a review course; it was not a learn-it-the-first-time course. But they were begging for help.

I didn't want to turn them away, but I also didn't want them to spend money to "review" when it appeared that they had not yet learned the information. By then, I was acutely aware of the difference between initial acquisition of knowledge, and retention of such knowledge. I searched for a framework, a strategy, methods, or even just some quick tips to help them, but found nothing. I knew there must be some way to figure out where they went wrong, and how to help them.

At some point several years later, I began to see patterns— the underpinnings of different candidates' failures. Then, by understanding the patterns of where they went wrong, I could articulate 3 Rs that can help people to pass on next try: Reflecting on both cognitive and affective strengths and weaknesses, identifying the reasons why an individual failed, and finally, regrouping.

The aim of this publication is to help you pass your multiple choice, comprehensive IBLCE exam on your very next try. You will be able to accomplish this goal if you follow my 3-step formula: reflect, reason, and regroup. I'll show you how.

Many famous artists, politicians, scientists, authors, entrepreneurs and others have failed miserably—and publicly—many times. Take heart in remembering that Walt Disney was fired from the local newspaper because he "lacked imagination and had no good ideas." Continue to take heart! Some of the most successful people you can name have probably had more than their share of failure. But they recovered from it, and were better for it! You can do the same.

Each year, about 500 people fail the IBLCE exam. Each year, I am more and more determined to help them. I've helped many people just like you to get the right tools in their toolbox. They've accepted my experienced and out-stretched hand; now I'm offering it to you.

Unit I: Reflect on What You Feel, Know and Do

Life moves fast. You might not feel inclined to take time to stop and reflect when the next endeavor is calling. Barreling ahead might work in some circumstances, such as after completing a project or celebrating a big success, but it doesn't work at all after a failure.

Reflection helps us to hit the "pause" button before we move full-steam ahead. By reflecting on what has happened, we can better understand ourselves, and we can figure out how to move forward. Otherwise, we run the serious risk of making the same mistakes with the same result: failure. When we stop to reflect on the current situation, we have a better shot at our goal: success.

In this unit, you'll have an opportunity to reflect on three things: How you feel, what you know, and how you do.

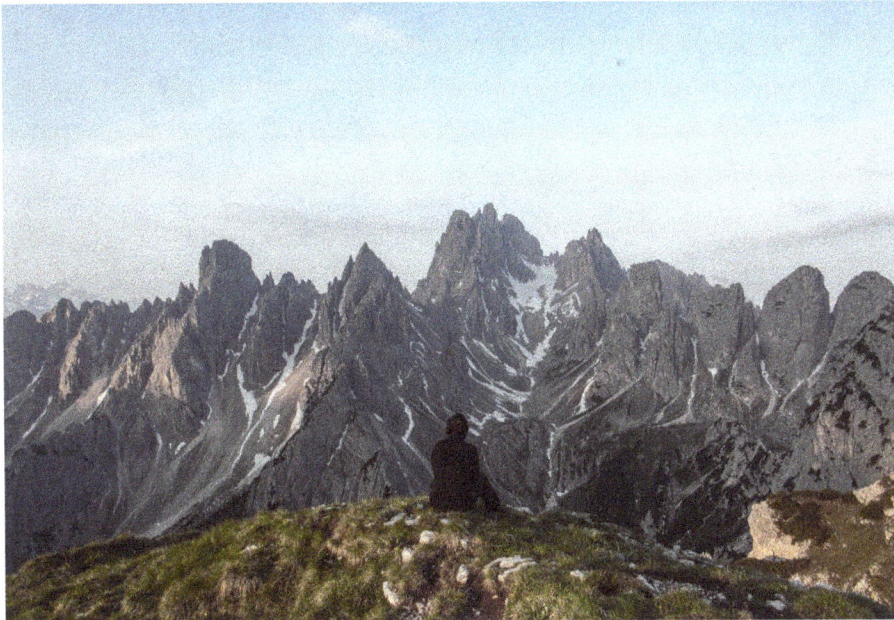

. . . .

1

Chapter 1: How You Feel About Taking Exams

Our emotions have a major role in all our endeavors. Consider, emotions are energy in motion. When you have negative energy, your "motion" will be towards a negative experience. By the same token, if you have positive energy, you will move towards a positive experience.

We see this in everyday events and experiences. Have you ever watched a basketball game and noticed a player who is just "hot"? Every shot from the floor, every shot under the basket, every shot from the foul line—the ball goes right straight through the basket. The more shots taken, the more points scored. It's as if he can't turn it off. He literally has energy in motion.

On the other hand, we've all had that day when things just didn't go well from the start. The alarm didn't go off when it was supposed to, traffic was horrible, you arrived late for work, you spilled coffee on your shirt, and everything just seemed to be in a downward spiral. Yes. Positive begets positive, and negative begets negative.

Research has shown that your attitude towards exam-taking is a major factor in determining your score. So, it's important to take a good hard look at how you feel about exams. And, if you've failed any exam, it's important to take a good look at how you view every aspect of the failure experience.

In this chapter, we'll talk about how you feel about failure in general, how you feel about failing an exam, and what timeframe you assign to failure.

Take a moment to reflect upon how you feel right now. Circle the word(s) that most closely describe your feelings about failing the exam.

Having failed this exam, I feel:

angry	determined
ashamed	disappointed
defeated	doubtful
deflated	dumb
devastated	foolish

frightened	sad
hopeless	silly
humiliated	surprised
incapable	trapped
indecisive	uncertain
insecure	unsettled
pressured	wiped out
relieved	other: _____
resentful	

How You Feel about the Outcomes of Failures

During my junior year of high school, I failed my New York State Regents Exam in Trigonometry—and hence, the course. Before my second attempt, an older student who was a National Merit Scholarship winner offered to help me. In addition to helping me with the exam's content, this smart kid recommended that I focus on test-taking strategies, too. This advice was instrumental to my success on retaking the Regents Exam, and expanded my thinking about areas of exam prep leading me to write, years later, *Test-Taking Strategies: A Guide to Taking and Passing the IBLCE Exam.*

Fortunately, I passed the trig exam, but more importantly, that smart kid later became my husband! Had I not failed trig the first time, I might not have met him. Sometimes, what seems to be a colossal failure is an opportunity to experience something much greater.

I've had other failures along the way, too. I miserably failed the Graduate Record Exam (GRE). In fact, I failed so badly that a representative of the exam's creator, Educational Testing Service (the parent of the GRE exam) company called me at home with my results. She explained, "Miss Biancuzzo, we have never had an examinee score so low since the exam was first administered in 1949. We felt your score must be a mistake, so, at no cost to you, we hand-scored your exam and that is indeed your score."

Great. Who knows? I may still hold the world's record for the lowest score ever on the GRE exam! In spite of the phone call I received, I determined that I would not be deterred from getting into the graduate school of my choice.

Instead, I spent some substantial time reflecting on what my preparation had been (very little) and my anxiety level during the exam itself (very high.) Once again, what seemed like a failure was an opportunity to learn. It sounds obvious now, but at the time, I needed to learn that hard lesson:

low preparation + high stress = failure

It's in part because of my own experiences with exam failure that I am so dedicated to helping others pass the exams they face. I have taught thousands of health care professionals so that they would be ready for the high-stakes, career-critical IBLCE exam—whether taking it for the first time, the second, or more. What is initially a failure can ultimately lead to a successful outcome.

How You Feel About Taking Exams

Few people relish the idea of having to take an exam. Yet most people would agree that they want professionals they rely on to have to pass exams to show they are qualified to safely or effectively do their jobs. Exams measure one's ability to safely do one's job, so exams are a good thing. Would any of us want to be on the road if no one had passed the driving exam? Would any of us want to be represented by a lawyer who hadn't had to pass the bar exam? And surely, none of us would want to undergo a surgical procedure at the hands of a surgeon who had not passed the medical board exam!

Similarly, breastfeeding mothers should be assured that the lactation professional they see is qualified for that work, as indicated by meeting the minimum requirements for exam eligibility and proving their expertise on the IBLCE exam.

But breastfeeding mothers and babies aren't the only ones who benefit from the IBLCE exam requirement. As an exam-taker, you too benefit.

Passing the exam can make you feel exuberant! Jubilant! Proud! Thrilled! Exhilarated! Empowered! That can be hard to believe when you've experienced a recent failure, but just wait. When you pass the exam, you will see. One IBLCE test-taker told me: "I love taking the IBLCE exam! I always look forward to beating my last score. Actually, I love taking all kinds of exams! Exams make me feel smart. When I get my results, I strut around for days patting myself on the back!" Is she just puffed up and conceited? No. She is self-assured and confident. She anticipates a big reward, and she gets it! Just seeing how well she can do (and achieving her personal best) is a big motivator for her.

Of course, not everyone looks forward to taking exams. Most people usually dread it. They take the exam only because they "have to" in order to earn some recognition or take advantage of some opportunity. Some IBLCE exam candidates tell me they have been learning about breastfeeding and lactation for years, such as in their work with mothers and babies in a hospital or pediatric practice. They have decided to take the IBLCE exam because they have realized that passing the IBLCE exam (and earning the IBCLC credential) is a necessary step in gaining recognition for their expertise.

True, the sense of dread about taking the exam may start months before exam day, but getting the results can be an exhilarating, life-changing moment. For many, passing the IBLCE exam launches a new career!

Most assuredly, there are any number of reasons why people may dread taking the IBLCE exam, or any other comprehensive exam. Regardless of the particular reason, there is one major key to reducing the dread: Moving toward your fear. You move towards your fear by taking charge of preparing for, studying for, and taking the exam.

How do you view exams? Do you feel that they are just a hurdle to jump? Do you understand how important they are as an indication of a professional's qualifications, especially in areas of health care? Do you look forward to exams as a way to show off—at least to yourself, or perhaps to others—how well you know your stuff? What words would you use to describe how you feel about taking exams?

How You Feel About the Permanence of Failure

Most of us have failures in our past. When we learn that we've failed, it's easy to feel trapped by the news. And, it's easy to feel certain that our dream for doing or being something will never come true. Not infrequently, we grieve for ourselves and our loss. It can seem as if we have lost something forever.

Even if you haven't failed an exam before, you've probably known the sting of failure sometime. Maybe you experienced the feeling from flunking the road portion of your driver's test the first time, or falling off a two-wheeled bicycle. But those experiences didn't stop you, did they? Odds are, you treated those experiences as mere speed bumps, not roadblocks, and certainly not as permanent detours. At some point, you decided to try again, perhaps many times, with success as your goal.

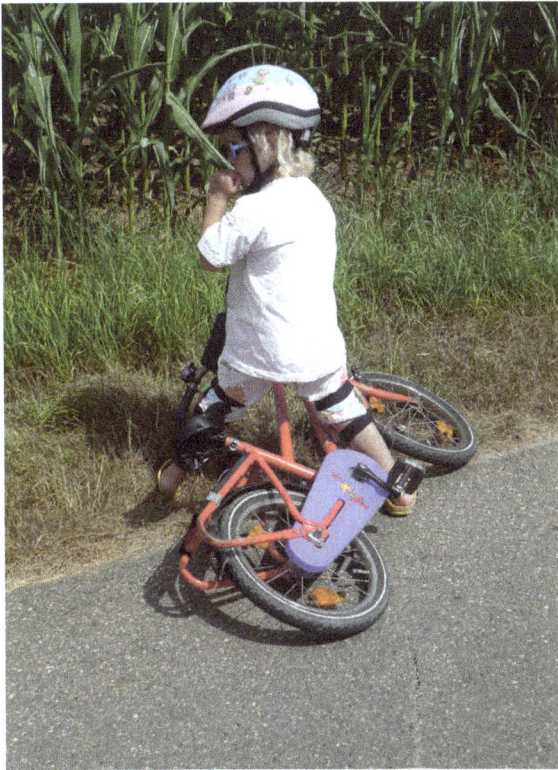

Failure certainly doesn't feel pleasant; disappointment isn't a feeling we like to carry around. Yet the most likely way to get through it is by allowing ourselves to feel those unpleasant, disappointing emotions. Remember, *emotion* is literally energy in motion! Often, that's what can provide the energy to taking the next step. As the saying goes, *we are driven to realize our goals by either inspiration or desperation*. So if you know that having your dream job depends on passing the IBLCE exam, you probably feel some desperation! That could be a good thing!

. . . .

7

Sure, the sting of failure is real. Plenty of people have tried and failed. You, too, have tried and failed. But failure is temporary. Failure is not permanent unless and until you say it is. The only difference between someone who fails and someone who succeeds is that the former allows the grinding halt of defeat, whereas the latter keeps moving forward with more resolve.

Which one will you be?

You already did a short exercise to identify how you felt about failing the exam.

Now, take a moment to think about moving forward? How do you feel about taking the exam in the future? Circle the word(s) that most closely describe how you feel about taking the IBLCE exam again.

anxious	helpless
doomed	in control
doubt	prepared
dread	uncertain
encouraged	unprepared
fearful	other: _____

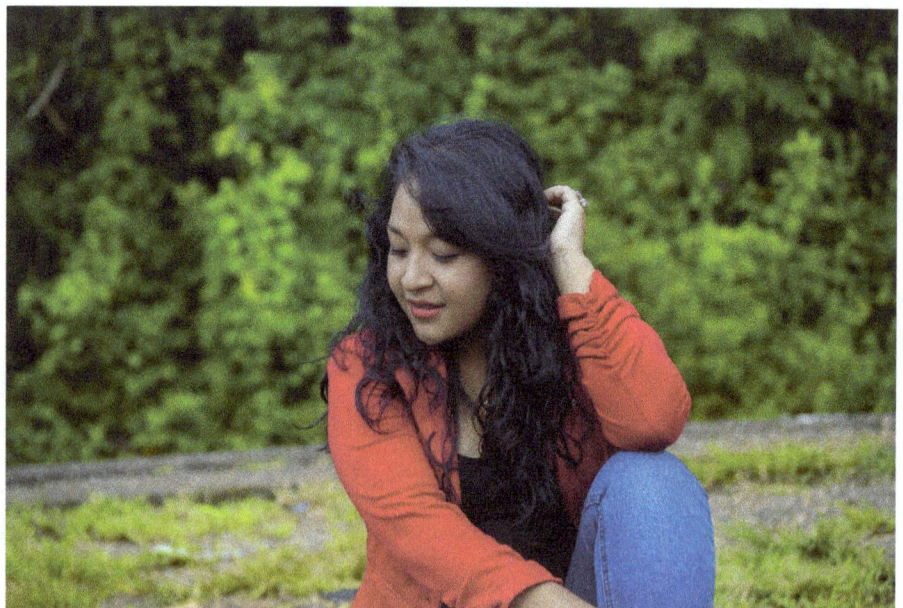

What's the Story In Your Head?

Some time ago, I was fortunate to host noted psychotherapist Sandra Reich on *Born to be Breastfed,* my weekly radio show for new mothers and those who care for them. Talking about anxiety, she used a phrase that gripped me: "the story in your head." Those five words summarized an entire body of scientific literature, as well as the symptom I've noticed in many of the IBLCE exam-takers I meet.

Sandra warned about the potential detriment of a negative story in your head, noting that it feeds a negative outcome. American industrialist Henry Ford made a similar observation many years ago, noting that "whether you think you can, or think you can't, you are right." In other words, if the story floating around in your head is "I'll fail" then indeed, you're probably right. Sandra Reich and Henry Ford are saying the same thing: Negative self-talk can be a self-fulfilling prophecy.

Such thinking ties to the popular science of neurocognition. One of the basic tenets is that what begins as "stories in your head" eventually is lived out by you—good or bad. In other words, if you are going around with anti-exam stories in your head, you are not ready for your next exam.

I've heard plenty of these stories from others and I've even heard some of these stories in my own head!

"I'm a terrible test-taker. I've always been a terrible test-taker. I just can't show what I know. I just can't."

"This is just too hard. I'm not smart enough. I don't know why I even signed up to take this exam when I'm just not smart enough to pass it."

"The IBLCE is out of touch! It's no wonder I can't pass this thing … these questions are irrelevant! IBLCE has it all wrong. It's their fault!"

"I don't see why I have to take this stinkin' test at all! I've been an IBCLC for 30 years. I know what I'm doing, and I shouldn't have to prove myself, over and over."

"I've already failed the IBLCE exam. If I failed it once, I will fail it again. I should just forget it, it's obvious I'm a failure."

"I'm too old to take a test. I'm 64 years old, and I haven't taken a test in more than 40 years. I just don't see how I can pass."

"The IBLCE exam is harder than the NCLEX exam. I didn't do all that well on the NCLEX, so I'm just doomed to fail the IBLCE exam."

"I just dread taking that IBLCE exam with all of their tricky questions. I hate that thing. None of those questions are relevant to my job, anyway."

But it's time to delete these negative stories, and replace them with positive ones.

For years, I had the "I'm a terrible test-taker" story in my head. Failing the Regents Exam in Trigonometry seemed to reinforce my self-doubt as test-taker. After that, I felt I had proof—*proof!*—that I was a terrible test-taker. Honestly, I had a tough time getting that negative story to disappear. I was unable to just wish it away but here's what I did: I replaced it with a positive story!

Called "positive affirmations," these positive stories always start with "I" or "I am." Instead of repeating, in my mind, "I'm a terrible test-taker," I would tell myself, "I am a good test-taker, and I will pass this exam with a very good score." If you can't wish away your negative story, try replacing it with a positive affirmation.

Some people think this is silly; they feel as if they are lying to themselves. But they are not. There's plenty of science to show that we become what or who we think about. People who have cut out a picture of their head and placed it on top of a slender body and hung it on the refrigerator have simply made a visual image of what they wish to become. They see themselves as slender, even though they are currently overweight. I repeat: We become what we think about. Whether you use words or the images, you create a positive story in our head so that you can have the self-fulfilling prophecy that has you celebrating rather than grieving.

Do you hear yourself repeating, over and over again, how much you hate exams? How unfair they seem? How unnecessary they are? How you feel too old to take an exam? Take a few minutes to write a paragraph or so about the story in your head.

Are you having trouble phrasing your own positive affirmations? Or maybe you feel silly doing positive affirmations? Okay, then try some of these insights, expressed by a variety of entrepreneurs, celebrities, and leaders over the years:

*They who have conquered doubt and fear have
conquered failure.*

—James Allen

*If you're not failing every now and again, it's a sign
you're not doing anything very innovative.*

—Woody Allen

*For every failure, there's an alternative course of action.
You just have to find it. When you come to a roadblock,
take a detour.*

–Mary Kay Ash

*A man can fail many times, but he isn't a failure until
he begins to blame somebody else.*

—John Burroughs

*Develop success from failures. Discouragement and
failure are two of the surest stepping stones to success.*

—Dale Carnegie

*Success consists of going from failure to failure without
loss of enthusiasm.*

—Winston Churchill

*Success depends upon previous preparation, and
without such preparation there is sure to be failure.*

—Confucius

*Our greatest weakness lies in giving up. The most certain
way to succeed is always to try just one more time.*

—Thomas A. Edison

*Do not fear mistakes. You will know failure. Continue to
reach out.*

—Benjamin Franklin

Every adversity, every failure, every heartache carries with it the seed of an equal or greater benefit.
—Napoleon Hill

Success seems to be connected with action. Successful people keep moving. They make mistakes, but they don't quit.
—Conrad Hilton

Failure is not a single, cataclysmic event. You don't fail overnight. Instead, failure is a few errors in judgment, repeated every day.
—Jim Rohn

You often pass failure on your way to success.
—Mickey Rooney

Failure is not fatal, but failure to change might be.
—John Wooden

The season of failure is the best time for sowing the seeds of success.
—Paramahansa Yogananda

If you learn from defeat, you haven't really lost.
—Zig Ziglar

Chapter 2: Reflect on What You Know

I would wager to say that most of us don't have a clear estimation how much knowledge we possess. We often focus on what we think we don't know. It's easy to get caught in a trap of thinking there are holes in our learning that we need to fix. That's okay; knowing what we don't know is good for self-improvement. But ruminating on holes in our knowledge base, or beating ourselves up about those holes, isn't helpful.

In truth, for taking the IBLCE exam (or any exam), what we need is to see ourselves and our abilities as they are: no better and no worse. And, we need to be able to contextualize that in a way that leads to success.

People who come to my exam prep courses are often eager to share their thoughts about what they do and do not know. Yet in many cases, they stumble when trying to articulate their learning needs in relation to the IBLCE exam. Sometimes, what they know is laudable! But it's highly unlikely to be something they'll see on the IBLCE exam. In other cases, they have a list of what they don't know and want to learn in the course—but those topics, too, are unlikely to be on the exam.

The real issue isn't about what you know, or what you don't know, in general. The issue is about what you need to know in order to pass the IBLCE exam!

In this chapter, we'll talk about how knowledge occurs in three different domains, and what this means for exam success.

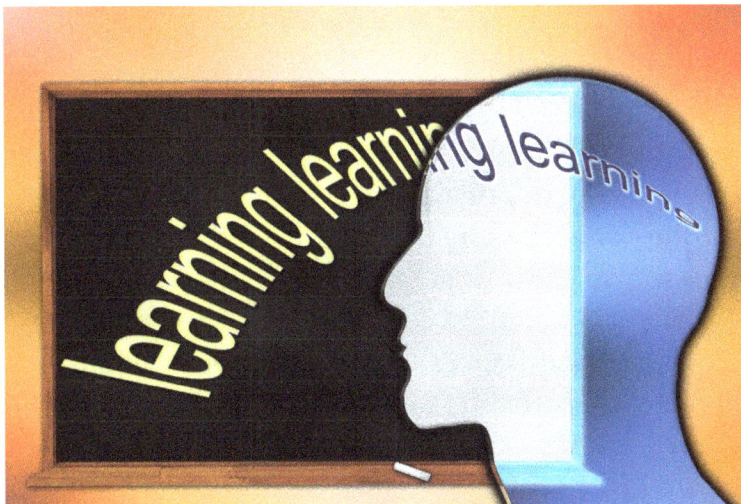

Cognitive Domain

In his seminal work in 1956, educational psychologist Dr. Benjamin Bloom showed that knowledge occurs in three different domains: cognitive, psychomotor, and affective. To pass a comprehensive exam such as the IBLCE, you'll need to learn in all three domains.

The *cognitive* domain has to do with mental abilities or knowledge. The theme is HEAD knowledge. The vast majority of questions on any high-stakes, career-critical exam test your abilities in the cognitive domain. Therefore, you should closely examine how well you've prepared.

Cognitive learning almost always involves some sort of formal course work. That is certainly the case for those who wish to be eligible to sit for the IBLCE exam. Candidates must have completed two major areas of study: The healthcare science education and the lactation-specific courses. If your cognitive learning isn't rock solid, you must revisit how, when and where you did your initial academic preparation.

Let's take the IBLCE's requirement for completion of the healthcare sciences courses. IBLCE doesn't care if you took your anatomy course 35 years ago, but you should care! If you've forgotten what a philtrim is, or what the incisive fossa is, or if you can't relate the amygdala to breastfeeding, maybe it's time to brush up a little—or hunker down a lot! You could do this on your own, or get minimal help, or, if needed, repeat your anatomy course.

Similarly, many IBLCE candidates have accumulated their 90 hours of lactation-focused education through a hodge-podge approach. Notice I said "accumulated" their hours. Accumulating hours of information is not the same as actually learning.

Do whatever is necessary to gain or review information you might need for the exam. (Be sure to review the ***IBLCE's Detailed Content Outline*** so you know what topics IBLCE has identified the exam covers.) But know that most cognitive-level questions on a comprehensive, high-stakes, career-critical exam are not simple recall questions. You will most certainly need to recall information to answer correctly, but the exam will require you to apply your recollection of the material to answer items that ask you to identify some specific action that would be appropriate.

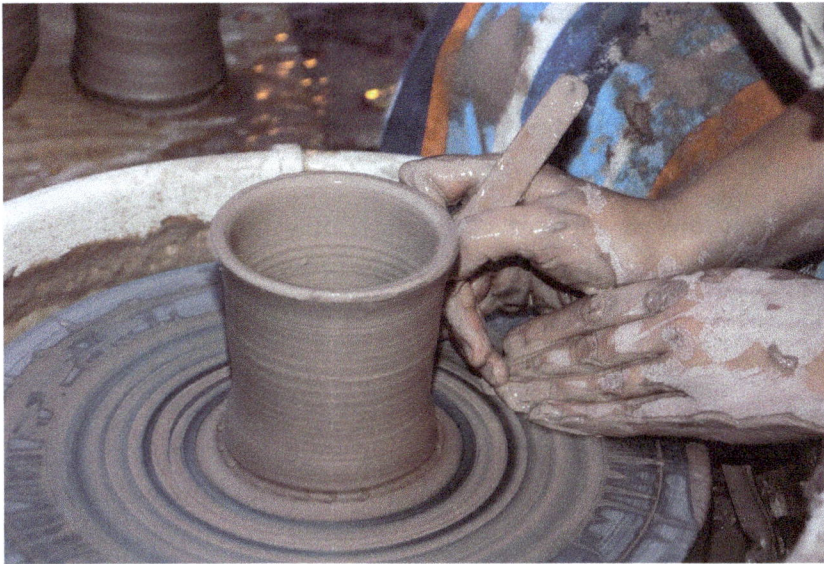

Psychomotor Domain

The psychomotor skills are those that involve manual or physical skills. The theme is knowing through your HANDS. No, the IBLCE exam won't ask you to actually pick up a piece of equipment and assemble or disassemble it. It certainly won't hand you a baby, or a mother's breast! However, I doubt that most people would be able to answer a test item about "hands" skills unless they had actually performed the skill at some point.

Here are some tasks in the psychomotor domain that I would consider fair game for the IBLCE exam to cover:

- teaching a mother how to hand express her milk
- estimating the amount of milk a mother would express and then selecting the best size container
- adjusting the height of a nursing supplementer to increase or decrease flow
- picking the first of many steps to assemble a piece of equipment
- calculating the volume of milk needed for a baby of a certain age.

As I've taught courses, I frequently mention a piece of equipment, such as a nursing supplementer, or some other device. Almost always, someone in the room says, "What is a [fill in the blank]?" I suppose it's possible to successfully answer an exam item having do with a piece of equipment you've never used; the exam is multiple-choice, so you could always guess. But you're more likely to get the right answer if you are responding from some hands-on experience.

Not all psychomotor questions are related to equipment, but certainly, equipment situations (and other hands-on techniques, such as hand expression) lend themselves to psychomotor questions.

If the psychomotor domain is harder for you, hands-on experience may be critical for your exam prep. Your ability to perform psychomotor tasks in "real life" is likely to predict how well you handle psychomotor questions on the exam. If you have trouble handling equipment in real life, you'll want to be sure to review your knowledge of it before the exam. At the very least, you will need to familiarize yourself with the relevant equipment or techniques.

Affective Domain

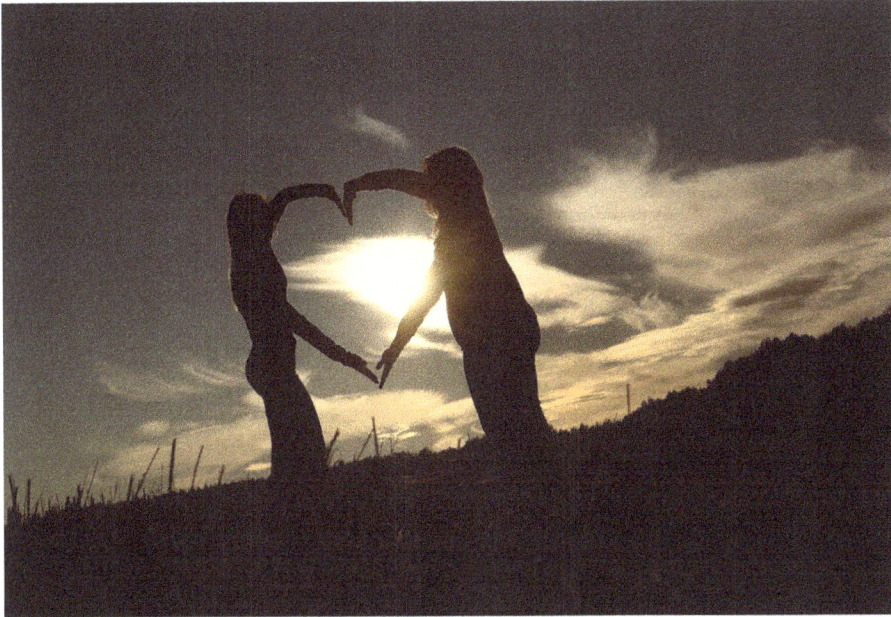

The affective domain, while while frequently ignored in teaching/learning, can be—and often is—integrated into comprehensive tests. The theme is knowing through the HEART. You might mistake these for cognitive-domain test items, but in truth, the items related to values and beliefs are actually testing your mastery in the affective domain.

Here are some tasks from the affective domain that I would consider fair game for the IBLCE exam:

- responding respectfully to a question from a gay couple
- selecting a culturally-appropriate visual aid for your prenatal class
- choosing an approach to persuade someone of the superiority of human milk over formula
- recognizing that a mother is too exhausted for a teaching session at this moment

Affective domain questions are about learning (or teaching) as related to human emotion.

Honestly, creating an affective-domain test item is difficult. You probably won't get many of these, but you can be almost sure that you will face at least a few.

Chapter 3: Reflect On What You Can Do: Exam Performance

No matter how you feel, and no matter how much you know, eventually, what it all comes down to is, what can you do on the exam? Before you rush into a high-stakes, career-critical exam, be sure you are ready. Here are some questions to ask yourself:

- Can I manage my time?
- Am I usually able to narrow down my answer to at least 2 options?
- How well have I performed on full-scale (175 question) practice exams that cover the entire *IBLCE Detailed Content Outline*
- How do I feel? How confident am I that I can pass successfully? Remember, a passing score not only reflects what you know but also your ability to believe in yourself and replace any negative inner stories with positive ones.
- Why are you taking this exam? Is it for a new job? For fun? For a sense of accomplishment? To show that you have one more credential than someone else?
- Did I really understand what was on this exam when I took it before? Or did I think, "Oh, I've been doing this sort of thing for years. I can surely pass an exam."
- What's the worst thing that could result from failing this exam again? Will I be fired from my job, or just disappointed in myself?
- What's the worst thing that could happen if you *don't* take the exam? Will waiting make a difference? Is this related to a job opening?

Some people are born ready! Others need to take some time before they wade into something. There is no shame in waiting if you're really not ready. The question is for you to understand the consequences of what might or might not happen if you delay.

The "Anatomy" of an Exam Item

Most certification or licensure exams, including the IBLCE exam, use a multiple-choice format. Before taking a multiple-choice exam, it's helpful to know the "anatomy" of the exam item. Most people just call this the "question." But actually, the question is only

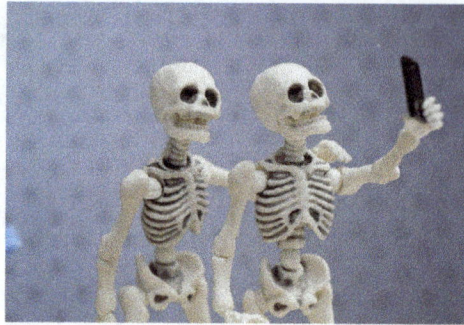

part of the item. In a multiple-choice test item, there is a stem and several options.

The stem is the first part of the test item. It contains the information on which the question is based. Stems come in two basic formats: (1) the simple question or (2) the partial sentence (i.e., sentence fragment). There are some variations.

Following the stem, there are several options. Usually, there are 4 options, but occasionally there are 3 or 5 options. Among these options, you'll find only one correct answer; the other options are called *distracters*. I like to remind exam-takers that there's a reason why experts call those options distractors. It's because they *distract* you from picking the right answer!

I have written an entire publication on *Test-Taking Strategies*, so I'm not going to belabor those points here. The purpose of this chapter is to have you reflect on your ability to perform on an exam. It is important that you know the basic "anatomy" of the exam first, and then you can reflect on your ability to truly look at the entire exam item, and read each word carefully.

I'd like to briefly address qualifiers: Qualifiers are those words that "qualify" the answer. Qualifiers are words such as best, least, most, first, last. How do you do with qualifiers? Here's an example.

Which of the following is the best utensil for eating yogurt?

a. knife

b. spoon

c. fork

Heaven knows, if you're clever and patient, you could load your yogurt onto a knife and eat it that way. I cheerfully admit that I've eaten yogurt with a fork when I've been on the road and that was the only utensil I had with me. But the best utensil for eating yogurt is, clearly, the spoon.

Do you see how focusing on the word "best" is the key to getting the right answer for this exam item? I've taught elementary, high school, undergraduate, graduate students, and those who are already licensed professionals. All of them have a tendency to overlook these qualifiers unless they really focus on them.

How do you think you do with these "qualifiers"?

Four Types of Headsets: Which One Is Yours?

I've seen many people who are seemingly capable of passing, and yet, they fail. They have perhaps even learned and retained the exam-related material. For one reason or another, they have what I call "headset" issues. I'm not an educational psychologist, but over many years of helping thousands of people, I have encountered four different types of headsets:

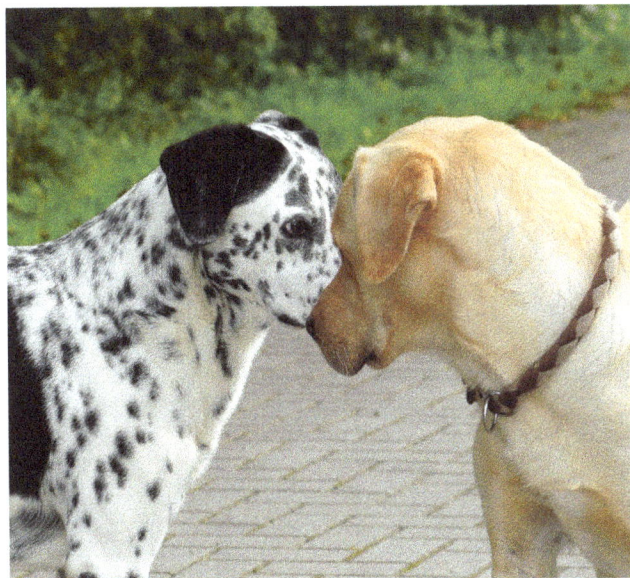

Under-focusers

Under-focusers are those who are focused on the exam at large, but not the exam item they are currently facing. Typically, this type of exam-taker focuses only on part of the question, or part of the options, but not the entire item or option.

Here's a very, very common mistake I see when I give a mock exam in my *Lactation Exam Review* course. Attendees pick an option that constitutes a true statement or a reasonable action, but that option did not answer the question.

Examinees will often complain that a question was "tricky." I disagree. If the question says, "which of the following actions is the IBCLC obligated to do" then the correct answer is the one that represents an *obligatory* action. The other actions may be good or helpful, but not obligatory.

Here are a few symptoms and characteristics I've noticed about under-focusers.

- Very quick to finish, possibly the first or one of the first few people to finish and leave the exam room. Is their speediness a symptom of being overconfident? Is their speed a symptom of their anxiety? I don't know. But I'm convinced there's a relationship between their high speed and low focus.
- History of being a high-achievers; they have a long history of doing well and do not perceive themselves as vulnerable on an exam.
- Gravitate towards main ideas rather than small details; more likely to take a "broad brush" approach to learning and communicating.

Of these "symptoms" the one I notice the most frequently is the speediness. And, interestingly, when we analyze results from the mock test, they often blurt out, "OH! I didn't notice the [whatever]. I knew that! I knew better! I don't know why I picked that other answer!" Ok, I know exactly why they picked the wrong answer! They overlooked the [whatever] word, which was the key word to selecting the right answer!

The question you need to ask yourself is: Are you an under-focuser?

Overthinkers

Over-thinkers are those test-takers who make the question harder than it actually is. I recognize these people immediately. Why so? Because I'm one of them!

I know I'm overthinking the question when I feel frustrated by a seeming lack of information. Often, I read an exam question and hear myself saying, "It depends on if..." I've learned to recognize that as a signal that I'm overthinking a question. If the answer truly depended on the information that I assume to be lacking, then the stem of the exam item would have given that piece of information.

I also know I'm overthinking when I talk myself out of the right answer. Distractors (the options that are wrong) can catapult me into having a distracting and destructive dialogue in my head. Let's say that the test item asks about a side effect of a particular drug. Before marking my answer, my inner dialogue goes like this:

> *"Oh, the correct answer is A. Yes, it's A. I learned that in first-year nursing school and I've seen it many times in clinical practice. For sure, it's A. No, wait. What about C? I've never read or heard or seen that, but yeah maybe C could be the drug's side effect. Maybe I'm out of date; maybe A is no longer a side effect, maybe there's some new side effect that I'm unaware of. I'm probably the only person in this room who doesn't know that C is a side effect ..."* With this dialogue in my head, I can talk myself out of the correct answer.

The next one is that I spend a lot of time trying to justify an option that simply isn't the answer! Or, I want to justify why another option should be the answer—but it's just not there! Or, I get hung up on the meaning or implication of a word in the stem or the options. (How *thorough* was that doctor's *thorough* assessment? How long ago did the client have that "earlier" injury?)

Some symptoms of the over-thinker are that they hear themselves thinking:

- "It depends on if…"
- "I don't like the word [fill in the blank]. That sounds too harsh."
- "At my hospital, we would never do it like that anyway!"
- "I wouldn't do any of those things. I would do something else!"
- "I marked A for the answer but actually, maybe B could be right, too…"
- And, in addition to their inner dialogue, typically, over-thinkers are:
- very conscientious students
- very experienced, and have both depth and breadth of knowledge
- often change their first-choice answer

- slow to finish, possibly being the last or one of the last people to finish an exam

The question you need to ask yourself is, am I an over-thinker?

Confidence-Lackers

Confidence Lackers are those people who simply lack confidence in themselves. Typically, they have a long history of being "bad test-takers" and hence, they are probably at higher risk for thinking that they will fail the next exam. Worse still, they continue to tell themselves that they are "bad test-takers" and so, it becomes a self-fulfilling prophesy. Again, I harken back Henry Ford's quote, "Whether you think you can or think you can't, you're right." Decades of research since then have shown that we can think ourselves into something, or think ourselves out of something. If you have gone into the exam thinking that you can't do it, you are already halfway to failure.

In my experience, here are the symptoms of the confidence-lackers:

- They have a long history of not doing well on exams.
- Some teacher or parent has told them that they are not good test-takers.
- They have "proof" through their own eyes, or through the eyes of their parents or teachers—and now believe they are not good test-takers.
- They don't tell me their test score when discussing their results—even though they know I'm the one who assigned them that score!
- They may have a more "irregular" academic record, perhaps doing well in some subjects or courses, but poorly in others.
- They spend a lot of time giving themselves negative affirmations, such as "I'm a bad test-taker." They tell others that line, too, as a way to somewhat "excuse" themselves in advance.
- They tend to take a long time finishing any exam.

Are you lacking in confidence? If so, you need to find a way to gain confidence. Lacking confidence will for sure affect your outcome.

Nervous Nellies

Nervous Nellies are those who are very anxious. They may be lacking in confidence, but their "symptom" is actually much bigger. They are so anxious that they simply cannot do their best on the exam. Again, I've seen these people when they are taking a 50-question mock exam in my Lactation Exam Review course. It's not even a real exam, and it has only a fraction of the number of question as on the "real" exam.

Nervous Nellies begin exhibiting anxious behaviors several hours before they face the mock exam. They are especially concerned about what happens to them if they score poorly. I assure them that they still get credit for completing the course, and other attendees will not know how well or how badly they scored.

Yet, they have a general sense of uneasiness, and they will sometimes continue to ask questions about "the test" throughout the morning, even though I don't give the mock exam until nearly noon. When we distribute the mock test, they begin asking questions about the mechanics of the test before everyone has received a copy. ("Do I need a pencil? What do I do if I change my mind about an answer?") As a result, they lose focus and work themselves into a tizzy.

The most blatant example of a Nervous Nellie I can think of was a woman who attended my course in Cleveland some time ago. She answered the first dozen or so questions on the mock exam, and then passed out. She was completely unable to finish. I later found out that she was diabetic. My guess is that she became so anxious that she quickly used up her circulating glucose. (And yes, the mock exam is before lunch.) Later, I told her I was so sorry she had had to experience this, but in a way, I was glad: It was a clear indication that she needed to reduce her anxiety, and bring a snack with her on the day of the exam.

Some symptoms of the Nervous Nellies are:

- early and continued expressions of fear and doubt about exam performance
- difficulty concentrating; focused on the outcome of the exam, rather than the process of taking it
- sweaty palms

. . . .

25

- trembling fingers
- shallow breathing
- increased pulse

The Nervous Nellies are often under-focusers because their anxiety level is so high. In essence, then, the Nervous Nellies can be experiencing a double-whammy when they go to take the exam.

Be honest with yourself: Are you a Nervous Nellie?

Now that you have reflected, and have a clearer idea of how your feelings impact your exam-taking experience, hold on tight! Next, you'll learn to reason through what's going on, and begin problem-solving in order to pass next time!

Unit II. Reason: Problem-Solve to Pass

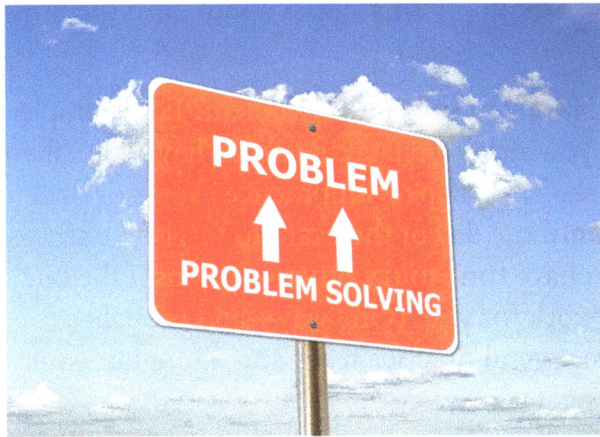

It's time to face facts: If you've failed the IBLCE exam, you have a problem. Fortunately, problems *can* be solved. But where to start? As Albert Einstein famously noted, "We can't solve problems by using the same kind of thinking we used when we created them." I recommend using a classic, 8-step problem-solving process to shake up our thinking and enhance our understanding of the problem, as well as identify possible solutions

Define the problem. What is the status quo? How does it need to change?

Gather data. What information can you find to substantiate the problem as it appears to be? This step involves finding facts and exploring feelings. Most people immediately recognize the importance of finding the facts related to the problem; few recognize the huge impact of how feelings can also affect exam results.

Analyze the data. What are the root causes of the existing problem? (Whereas Step 2 focuses on developing a list or a description, this step is more of an analysis of the information you gathered.)

Generate possible solutions. Brainstorm any and every possible option that might fix the problem, without worrying about feasibility (yet!) This step is about *generating ideas*.

Select a solution. Consider all the possible solutions, weighing their costs and benefits, as well as their likelihood for success. Select one (or a few) that are workable. This step is about planning for action.

Plan and implement. Think about what you must have to "do" your chosen selection. Then, do it! This step is about both planning and acting.

Re-visit the problem. Have you solved the problem? For example, if your problem is that you lacked test-taking skills, have you taken steps to develop those skills, perhaps with practice exams or drill questions? Don't wait until the day of the exam to re-visit your problem! You'll want to have time to try other solutions if the one you first chose doesn't work for you. (One way—and probably the best way—is to take several practice tests, and figure out your strengths and weaknesses.)

Continue to improve. In some ways, test-taking is no different than learning to ride a bicycle. You may fall off the bicycle when you first try to ride. But if you keep at it, you'll eventually gain the confidence, knowledge, and skills to succeed. That's the same with the IBLCE exam.

In this unit, we'll walk through each of these steps.

Chapter 4: Define the Problem and Gather Data

Frankly, no one wants to have a problem. When we do, it's a sure thing we want it solved sooner rather than later. The "sooner" will occur when you can clearly state the problem. As Charles Kettering, the famous U.S. inventor and long-time head of research for General Motors, insisted: "A problem well stated is a problem half-solved."

At first, it seems tempting to say that the problem is glaringly obvious: You failed the exam! So, isn't the problem "how to deal with the failure"? Actually, no. The problem is, "how to pass the IBLCE exam *on the very next attempt.*"

I suppose everyone has a favorite approach to use when faced with a problem. Personally, I favor Lewin's Change Theory model when I need to solve a problem. Developed by social psychologist Kurt Lewin, the basis for the model is recognizing the need to figure out how to get from the current (or "problem") state to your desired state (or "solution"). If you're reading this book, that means getting from not having your IBCLC certification to earning it.

Here, we'll start with analyzing the data, and go through the problem-solving process.

Over the years, I have helped thousands of people to prepare for and pass their IBLCE exam. During that time, I've noticed patterns of common problems. Here, I'll identify the four top problems, as well as solutions that might help you to move towards success the next time you take the IBLCE exam.

Inadequate Mastery of Vocabulary

I cannot overemphasize the importance of knowing the vocabulary that is relevant to your field of study. *Unquestionably*, reading is directly related to preparation for and performance on a comprehensive exam. Vocabulary is an essential element of reading comprehension. Unless you have mastered the vocabulary of this discipline you cannot fully comprehend the material you are studying, or being tested on.

Vocabulary is the foundation for understanding

When I was in grade school, textbook chapters started with a list of vocabulary words. Students were expected to learn the vocabulary words before they launched into full-blown study of subject matter. Any good teacher knows that students need to learn basic relevant vocabulary or facts before they can master concepts or materials that use them.

In adulthood, we are rarely, if ever, tested on word definitions. But professional exams do test on the broader ideas associated with a subject-specific vocabulary. We might be asked to explain phenomena associated with that word. We might need to take an action associated with that word. If we don't know what the word means, we're sunk before we start.

Before re-taking the IBLCE exam, make sure you have a good understanding of the vocabulary of lactation practice. Don't get caught by words that are more technical (like distal, seroconversion, acrocyanosis, Bauer's reflex, leptin, lipophilic, and many more). A clear understanding of a word is important for both studying and test-taking.

Without an understanding of the vocabulary (including technical and non-technical terms), test-takers cannot form what might be called "cognitive connections." Although they may be able to read or say the words, they are not able to connect those words to other words or concepts, explain the implications of those words, or recommend action based on those words. In short, they won't do well on an exam that tests their knowledge of such implications or actions.

While studying, it can be tempting to skip over unfamiliar words. You might not think that such a word is important, and in some cases, it won't be! But the word is part of the bigger concept. Don't skip the words; learn them.

Fluency in English

It's important to be fluent in the language in which you are testing. In my experience, taking the exam in English can be a problem for many candidates who opt to do so even though it is not their first language. I have observed that the better the candidate can

. . . .

© 2017 Gold Standard Publishing

30

write in English, the less of a problem it seems to be during the exam; perhaps this reflects a better ability to make those "cognitive connections." I always encourage people to take the exam in their native language. The IBLCE makes the exam available in about 20 different languages each year!

Fluency in Medicalese!

It's all Greek

A α	B β	Γ γ	Δ δ
E ε	Z ζ	Θ θ	H η
I ι	K κ	Λ λ	M μ
N ν	Ξ ξ	O o	Π π
P ρ	Σ σ ς	T τ	Y υ
Φ φ	X χ	Ψ ψ	Ω ω

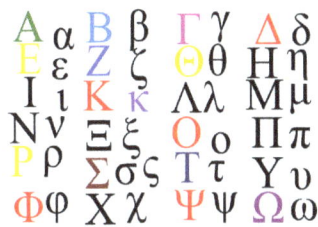

Most medical words are derived from Greek or Latin. Even candidates with English as their first language can have language problems when taking the IBLCE exam. Exam candidates who cannot define the words—technical or non-technical words—cannot demonstrate cognitive connections. They can read or say the words, but unless they can connect those words to other words or concepts, explain the implications of those words, or take an action based on those words, they won't do well on an exam that tests their knowledge of such implications or actions.

I have seen native English-speakers who don't have a complete understanding of the words they are reading, but the people who struggle the most are those for whom English is not their first language In either case, the result is about the same: They cannot make that cognitive connection.

Here's an example of a sentence I read earlier this morning:

> *"Nutritional status can influence epigenetic profiles by DNA methylation and histone modification."*

I need to stop and ask myself, if I actually know what that sentence means. I have a shallow understanding of what the word "epigenetic" means, but I don't really know what an epigenetic profile is. From my high school biology course, I know that DNA is genetic material, but luckily, I think I understand the word "gene." I more or less know the meaning of the word "methylation" and "histone". But I don't really know.

Unless I look up the words I don't know, I walk away with the understanding that nutritional status has something to do with genetic material that is modified in some way. But I really don't know what I just read. In fact, I don't even know if the sentence is saying that this thing—this event or whatever it is—is good or bad.

Few or Weak Connections of New and Old Information

Decades ago, the education gurus revealed that we learn best by connecting new information to information that we've already mastered. In truth, some teachers are very good at helping learners to bridge that gap between the known to the unknown; other teachers aren't good at it.

If you cannot adequately connect new information to old information, you will not do well on any comprehensive exam.

Results Revealed in IBLCE's Analysis

All candidates receive a computerized printout of their performance in the disciplines and chronological areas. Look at your report carefully. This could be your most valuable tool to analyzing where you went wrong, and why.

Your exam results report included indicators of your performance in the various disciplines and chronological areas covered by the IBLCE exam.

IBLCE's exam report has changed over the years. In 2016, the categories were updated to reflect those of the latest Detailed Content Outline. So if you took the exam between 1985 and 2015, those reports are different. But the principle for gathering the data you need is the same: Look at the disciplines and the chronological areas, and see where you had low scores.

Below is the real report received by an IBLCE exam-taker. This report was for her third unsuccessful attempt at passing the IBLCE exam, and she shared it with my staff and I when she called for "help!"

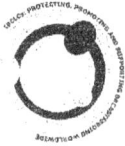

IBLCE
International Board of
Lactation Consultant Examiners

Score Report for the 2016 Examination

Total Score: 114.00
Minimum Passing Score: 128
Pass or Fail: Fail

Content Outline Area Subscores for Each Discipline and Chronological Period

Category 1	Points
CHRONOLOGICAL PERIOD	**114.00 of 175.00**
01. PRENATAL	12.00 of 18.00
02. LABOR/BIRTH	5.00 of 9.00
03. PREMATURITY	4.00 of 8.00
04. 0-2 DAYS	12.00 of 18.00
05. 3-14 DAYS	17.00 of 27.00
06. 15-28 DAYS	9.00 of 14.00
07. 1-3 MONTHS	12.00 of 19.00
08. 4-6 MONTHS	5.00 of 9.00
09. 7-12 MONTHS	3.00 of 4.00
10. BEYOND 12 MONTHS	3.00 of 4.00
11. GEN PRINCIPLES	32.00 of 45.00
SUMMARY:	**114.00 of 175.00**

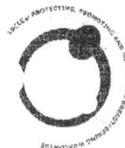

IBLCE
International Board of
Lactation Consultant Examiners

Score Report for the 2016 Examination

Total Score: 114.00
Minimum Passing Score: 128
Pass or Fail: Fail

Content Outline Area Subscores for Each Discipline and Chronological Period

Objective	Points
DISCIPLINE	**114.00 of 175.00**
I. DEV/NUTRITION	18.00 of 26.00
II. PHYS/ENDO	13.00 of 24.00
III. PATHOLOGY	19.00 of 31.00
IV. PHARMA/TOX	8.00 of 13.00
V. PSYCH/SOC/ANTHRO	17.00 of 21.00
VI. TECHNIQUES	20.00 of 25.00
VII. CLINICAL SKILLS	19.00 of 35.00
SUMMARY:	**114.00 of 175.00**

This exam-taker was new to us, so we asked her for a full history of her exam prep, including how she acquired the 90 hours of lactation-specific education (she used the hodge-podge approach), how long ago she had completed her required health sciences courses, and her recent and non-recent clinical experience.

We looked carefully at her subscores for the discipline, and the chronological areas. As you can see, she was weak in nearly every subscore. We recommended that she take a comprehensive 90-hour course.

Another person who contacted us for help in preparing to re-take the exam found herself in a different situation. She had fairly good subscores overall, with one glaring exception—the pharmacology/toxicology section. Her score led us to suggest completion of a topic-specific course, such as one we offer in Tough Topics. Since she wasn't a nurse, she had limited opportunity to gain the pharmacology/toxicology knowledge in the preferred way, through experience.

Accumulation of 90 Lactation-Focused Hours

Without a doubt, taking a comprehensive course is your best strategy for passing the IBLCE exam. It only makes sense: If you're preparing for a comprehensive exam, your best bet is to take a comprehensive course! I teach such a course, and there are others available as well.

In my opinion, anyone who does not take a comprehensive lactation course is gambling with their ability to pass the exam! To effectively move towards your desired state—passing—you must know your current state. It's as simple as that.

Chapter 5: Analyze the Data and Root Causes for Failure

I've looked in the fields of education, psychology, and business to find an organized framework for diagnosing or "analyzing" the data and root causes about failing a comprehensive certification or licensure exam. There is no such thing. I've had to develop my own model. After having helped many, many exam candidates, I believe that all exam failure can be attributed to one or more of the five reasons I've noted.

You weren't exposed to the content.

Being exposed to the right content is the first and most critical aspect of passing any exam. But how can you make sure you do this?

Certainly, a good first step is to review IBLCE's Detailed Content Outline. But honestly, I've never met any exam candidate who could look at that outline and clearly tell me the exact content they need to study.

What's more, most aspiring IBCLCs collect their 90 lactation-focused hours here and there, going to a conference on whatever topic du jour catches their attention, or is convenient to attend. Most focus on the "90 hours" requirement. Maybe you did, too. It's easy to let the "90" distract from the fact that it's supposed to represent learning about the many different topics that will be on the exam.

With no previous exam experience, and no expert guidance, how could you possibly study the topics that are likely to appear on the exam? How could any candidate prepare to pass a comprehensive exam without taking a comprehensive course?

When I first taught my *Comprehensive Lactation Course* in 2009, I spent about 100 hours planning the course, to ensure it covered IBLCE's outline. I'm talking about just *planning* the course; that doesn't include making slides or handouts, or delivering the course! IBLCE has revised its outline since then, and I keep updating my course to make sure it covers the topics the exam will cover.

You didn't understand the content.

Being exposed to the exam topics isn't enough. You also need to be able to make sense of the material in a meaningful way.

Once you've been exposed to the topics, you may be able to re-state, list, recognize, describe, and identify simple facts and concepts. But if you can't relate that content to your prior learning, explain it to someone else, or summarize it in your own words, then you don't fully understand it.

A great way to come to understand material is to write out a relationship, an explanation, or a summary. I believe Dawson Trotman's quote: *Thoughts disentangle themselves when they pass through the lips and fingertips.*

You didn't retain the content.

Maybe you were exposed to the right topics and understood everything right away. If you studied early, then gave it up sure that you were ready, you were probably surprised by your low score. Unless you can recall it, you're doomed to a low exam score.

Research in the education field has shown over and over that people do not retain information when they simply watch a video or hear a lecture. Don't be fooled by the claim that "adult learning principles" means having great photos. Seeing a video, looking at photos, or hearing a lecture doesn't automatically create an effective learning experience.

What does result in information retention is to actively participate in your learning experience. Don't take my word for it; ask those who have taken my courses. I hear it all the time. (Active learning is harder with an online-only program, but if an in-person course isn't possible for you, you can still find ways to do active learning.)

You couldn't apply the content.

Maybe retaining the relevant facts, concepts, or principles wasn't the problem. Could you apply the content to answer to exam items?

Sometimes when I teach, I direct learners to put their pens down, stop memorizing, and just listen. I want them to grasp the clinical "so-what." The IBLCE exam will present you with short vignettes.

Unless you understand how various circumstances affect the "memorized" information, you'll have trouble passing the exam.

Here is an example of a simple recall question:

Which of these speeds, stated in miles per hour, is the typical limit on many or most U.S. Interstate highways?

A.   35-40

B.   45-50

C.   55-60

D.   65-70

E.   75-80

Of course, you know that the answer is D, 65-70 miles per hour. This is a simple recall question. You either know it, or you don't.

Recall, although necessary, is not sufficient to answer an application-level question. Here is a question that is more akin to a clinical vignette:

Marie is an experienced driver. She has a late-model car, and is driving on Interstate 95, north to Baltimore. During her trip, snow begins falling at a rate of about two inches per hour. What is the highest speed Marie should be driving?

A.   45-50

B.   55-60

C.   65-70

Here, simply recalling that most speed limits on an Interstate Highway are 65-70 would not be adequate for answering the question. You would also need to know that snowfall of two inches per hour is a lot. (At that rate, a foot of snow would drop within six hours!) Generally, application-type questions require the candidate to use several facts to come to some kind of judgment, recommendation, decision, or similar action. And, if you had grown up in a snow belt (as I did!) having experience helps you to answer the question.

To prepare yourself for the exam, get clinical experience, and plenty of it, in a variety of settings with a variety of clients in a variety of circumstances. When you've gained knowledge with real-life mothers and babies, you can draw on it when you're faced with exam mothers and babies!

You couldn't perform.

You were exposed to the material, understood it, remembered it, and could apply it in the clinical area. But you didn't get the right answers on the exam—at least not often enough to pass. What happened?

Often, it seems to come down to what item-writers call "distractors." Remember, there's a reason why item-writers call those other options "distractors." It's because these options that distract you from picking the right answer! Developing good Test-Taking Strategies may be key for your success.

Or, it may be a problem of testing anxiety. That's common! Try our *Self-hypnosis CD*. Whether it works or not, let me know.

All the exam gurus insist that **your headset is a major determinant in your exam score**. It may sound corny, but never underestimate the importance of a positive mindset on the day of the exam.

The IBLCE exam is a career-critical, high-stakes exam. Even if you passed, you can learn how to do better by learning where your preparation could have been stronger.

Chapter 6: Generate Possible Solutions

To generate possible solutions to your problem, you need to have a clear analysis of data you have collected about your past experiences: your feelings about failure, your knowledge and methods for gaining information that is likely to be on the exam, and the extent of your clinical experiences. And, you'll need to do a little self-reflection: Is your problem due to one or more of the root causes we've explored? Is it related to knowledge exposure, comprehension, retention, application, or performance?

Earlier, I said that the problem is not that you failed the exam. The real problem is figuring out a way to pass the exam the next time. A major factor in all of this is the time it will take you to implement whatever solution or solutions you choose. Here are my suggestions:

1) **Pause.** Take some time to reflect upon your goals. This is your dream, and just as we cannot dream five minutes after we wake up, some of us cannot take an exam five months after we fail. It's okay to give yourself some time before jumping back in. However, the time taken should be the pause that refreshes your dream; it should not be the procrastination that destroys it.

 2) **Make a list.** Write down whatever you did to prepare for the exam the first time. Include the three universal requirements: completion of the health sciences courses, completion of your 90 lactation-specific hours, and your hours of clinical experience. Be sure to note the pros and cons of how each of those experiences prepared you for the exam.

3) **Consider your options.** Write down your different options for exam preparation. For example, if you took an online course last time, a different option would be taking a face-to-face course. If you did all of your clinical experience in hospital inpatient units, a different option would be working in the outpatient department. Make a list of the pros and cons of how you believe each of those experiences would prepare you for the exam.

4) **Be ready to get to the root of the problem.** Remember that in almost all cases, you need to find a solution to overcoming your root causes of failure: exposure, comprehension, retention, application, and performance.

Are you starting to feel ready to tackle this problem head-on? Take another look at your list of options. It's important to figure out which will work best for you. Then, you'll need a good plan for implementing them. To develop a solid, workable plan that will suit your needs, you take a few minutes to write the answers to the four above-mentioned considerations.

Chapter 7: Plan and Implement Best Solutions

Once you have generated several options, it's important to figure out which option or options will work best for you. Then, having found the best options, you'll need a good plan for implementing them. To get a solid, workable plan, you should write the answers to these questions:

Why do I want to pass the IBLCE exam? Why do I need this certification? Is it to keep my current job? To get a better hourly wage or a better salary in my current job? To get a better job or a different job? For a sense of achievement? To gain the respect of those who do not always acknowledge my talents? Remember, emotion is energy in motion. You will have more energy behind this effort if you are clear on why you are pursing the credential.

What are my learning needs? What is it I haven't learned that I should learn, or what is it that I am unable to do that I need to do in order to deliver high-quality care and/or pass the exam?

What and where are my learning resources? Do I have good computer access? Do I have the books I need? Have I identified the people or courses that can help me?

How can I get the time I need for exam prep? What will I need to do to convince my boss or my family that I need to devote time to doing whatever it is I need to do in order to pass?

What kind of situation works best for me? Do I need to be home with my kids to have the peace of mind that that they are tucked safely into bed when I begin my studying? Or do I need to get away from my place of employment, my colleagues, or my family so that I can hunker down and immerse myself in an intensive study session? (I have been astonished at the number of people who have used the words "escape" and "immerse" to describe their need for studying.) Is there some middle ground? Could I take my mother and my children with me and let them play while I settle down into an all-day course? If I'm home or at the office, do I need a set of earplugs? What do I need to succeed in my studying efforts?

What kind of financial resources will it take? How will I buy more books or enroll in a course or pay the IBLCE? What will it cost for travel and childcare?

Answering these questions will ensure you have a better understanding of what solutions will work for you. We'll talk more about implementing your plan in the next unit.

Chapter 8: Re-evaluate and Continue Improving

The key to re-evaluating your needs, your study strategies, and your accomplishments can be summarized with one word: Feedback! And, if you are working with a mentor or a course instructor, she will give you feedback. But if not, well, you need to find another way to get such feedback.

Most people find that the process of exam prep is improved by gaining feedback. From whom? It could be an experienced colleague, a mentor or a course instructor, if you have one. But what you want is another seasoned perspective on your approach to the IBLCE exam to help ensure you're set on the path to success.

From time to time, I ask people who come to my Comprehensive Course and my Lactation Exam Review courses: "What brought you here today? Why did you decide to come?" I've heard many reasons, but one that's stuck with me was from a participant who said: "I've already failed the exam twice. I started going through my books again, and my husband said, 'The last two times, you studied with yourself. This time, you should study with Marie.'"

I was intrigued by the phrase, "studied with yourself." She said, "with." The phrase "by myself" connotes studying alone. But the phrase "with myself" implies that she and her alter-ego were studying together.

The term alter-ego, a phrase first coined by Cicero in the first century Rome, means "a second self; a trusted friend." I do believe that studying with your second self, your trusted friend, can be an effective means of providing feedback! But do not mistake false reassurance or self-blame for giving you feedback about your mastery of the material.

Whether you provide feedback to yourself or someone else, you need to know the difference between praise, criticism, and feedback. Author and inspirational speaker Marty Brounstein makes this distinction well.

According to Brounstein, constructive feedback is "information-specific, issue-focused, and based on observation." However, "praise and criticisms are personal judgements about a performance or outcome." Here are some examples that you might be telling yourself as you study for the IBLCE exam:

- Praise: "Sally, you did a good job studying for the IBLCE exam today. You worked hard."
- Criticism: "Sally, you did a lousy job of listening to that webcast on hormones. You know you'll never be able to answer questions on that stuff."
- Positive feedback: "Sally, you tackled three of those matching exercises that Marie gave on hormones, and you got 100% of the first two right, and 85% of the last one right."
- Negative feedback: "Sally, you still can't name all of those hormones, or what function they perform, or even where they are. You didn't even try to tackle those matching exercises that Marie gave in the homework. And, at a gut level, you don't feel confident."

If you are not enrolled in a course, it will be much more difficult to give yourself feedback. And, if are you just reading and re-reading information, it will be almost impossible to give yourself constructive feedback. However, here are some examples of ways to provide feedback for yourself if you are reading a chapter in a book:

- **Define vocabulary words.** These may be presented at the start of the chapter, or you may need to find them (often italicized) in the text. Either way, force yourself to speak each word aloud, and state a definition for each in your own words. (After all, studies have shown that "talking to yourself" can be an effective way of helping you to remember information you need!) You can then give yourself feedback about how many you have correctly answered, and which ones were impossible for you. Note how many there are.
- **Draw a mind map.** Let's say the topic is mastitis. You could start by drawing "branches" for definition, associated pathological organisms, risk factors, signs and symptoms, treatments (including commonly-prescribed medications) and priorities for maintaining milk supply, and related teaching responsibilities. Provide positive or negative feedback for yourself, based on whether or not you could complete the mind map.

- **Use the technique of recitation.** It's simple to use, costs nothing, and is hugely effective. If done correctly, it provides almost immediate, accurate feedback!
- **Identify new learning.** Write down at least 10 new things you learned from the chapter. If you did not learn 10 new things, is it because you already knew most of what was covered in the chapter?

For some people, self-feedback works well. For those who come to my exam prep courses, feedback from a seasoned instructor can be invaluable. Clear and accurate feedback received from someone who is well-versed on the IBLCE exam helps to ensure you aren't just putting in time, but that your studying is focused on moving you towards your goal.

Now, you have made some serious inroads into problem-solving. But thinking it through, and making it happen are two different things! In the next unit, you'll learn how to re-group, and manage your resources.

Unit III: Re-Group: Manage Your Resources

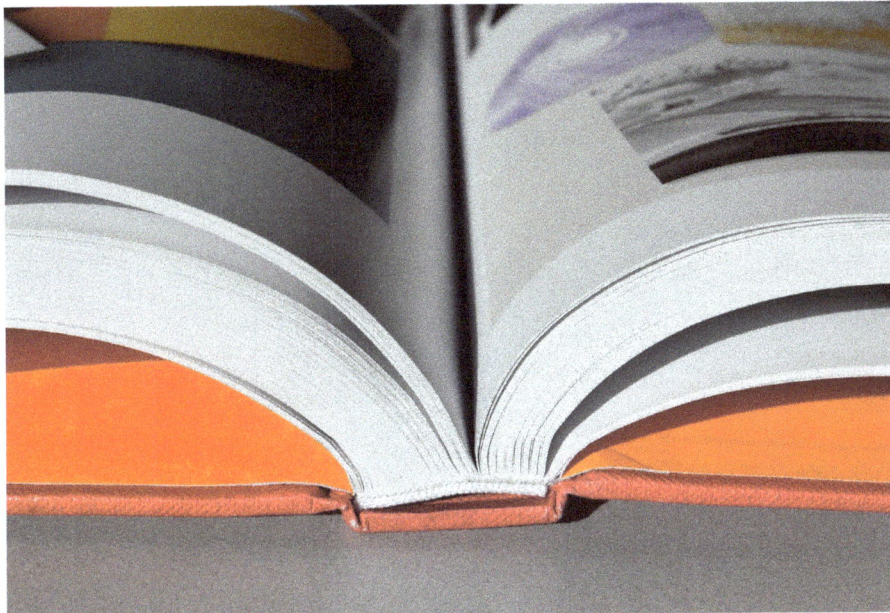

All of us wish for more and better resources. We often feel sure that if we had more books, better videos, more knowledgeable teachers, more money, or faster computers, all would be well in our world and our exam-taking endeavors. And, of course, more time! We all complain that we don't have enough time to prepare for the upcoming exam!

The thing is, though, that we will probably never have all the resources that we could imagine or wish for. And for sure, we will never have more than 24 hours in a day! So the trick, really, is not having more or better resources, but managing the resources we already have.

In this unit, you'll see how to embrace structure, plan a process to prepare for the exam, master test-taking strategies, and consider some resources you now have but perhaps haven't used. Most of all, you'll learn how to use your most precious resource—your time—in ways that you might never have before. I'll give you some very concrete ideas, because I truly believe it's not about *having* more; it's about *doing* more with what you have.

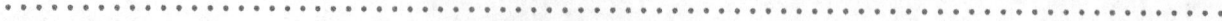

Chapter 9: Embrace Structure

As Pulitzer-prize winning author Charles Duhigg observed, "if you pose things in abstract, goal-related terms, it's much less likely that you will accomplish [the goal] than if you structure it as an actual activity." Duhigg is not diminishing the importance of goal-setting; many research studies have established the usefulness of goal-setting. Rather, he is saying that without an actual plan of steps to reach the goal, success is unlikely. In short, we all need structure to accomplish our goals!

"Structure" here is a plan for the arrangement of complex steps. Structures have defined boundaries. The elements are usually unchanging, and are related to one another. Structure gives form and stability to the whole.

Think of structure setting a framework for your success. While it's great to have a lofty goal—"I want to get my IBCLC so I can help mothers and babies breastfeed"— a structured plan must be used to make that a reality. Your plan should include all the actions you need to take along the way, as these support your dream.

In this chapter, we'll talk about the structure that supports your plan to pass the IBLCE exam. Generally, this includes: time management ("when": deadlines and calendars), resources ("what you need": material and equipment) and environment ("where": study location).

Deal with Deadlines: Take Control Where You Can!

"Time is free, but it's priceless. You can't own it, but you can use it. You can't keep it, but you can spend it. Once you've lost it, you can never get it back," notes Minnesota businessman Harvey Mackay.

Finding Time, or Managing Your Time?

We often talk about "finding" time, as though it is a buried treasure, a lost set of car keys, or an item that somehow sprouted legs and walked away! But we all have time. And, interestingly, each of us has exactly the same amount of time as anyone else. You and I don't have any more time in a day than Bill Gates, Stephen King, or the President of the United States. But they have world-class recognition, and we don't. Why? Because they knew it wasn't about "finding" time. It's about managing time.

Most highly successful people have simply managed to use their time more effectively than the rest of us. Highly successful people manage their time in a way that consistently produces results. But so can we! Time management is simply a skill to be learned.

Becoming aware of your time management skills is critical, not only as you prepare for the upcoming exam, but in your career, and your personal life, too. I know online surveys are a dime a dozen, but here's one that can help you gain tremendous insight into how you manage your time.[1] Taking 10 minutes or so to do this brief exercise will probably help you save hours of wasted time.

Identifying Important Dates

In many cases, you aren't the one setting the deadlines. Some external party has established the dates by which you must complete your requirements, submit your application, and be ready to take the test. But even though you had little say-so in setting the deadlines, you must deal with them. At the very least, you will need to know the deadlines, so that you don't miss applying for—or taking the exam!

What can you control about the deadlines? How much time you use to prepare to meet them. You need to figure out how much time you can realistically allot to exam prep. To do that, ask yourself these seven questions, and write down your answers.

- When must I submit my application for the exam?
- What is the date for the exam?
- How much time do I have between now and the exam dates?
- Between now and the exam date, what pressing commitments or priorities will also need my time?
- Are there days that I know I will be completely unable to do any preparation for the exam? (For example, your daughter's wedding day will keep you busy from dawn until dusk—and beyond!)
- Are there small pockets of time I can use for short, focused study? (Examples: time spent waiting for your son to finish

---

1   _http://psychologytoday.tests.psychtests.com/ take_test.php?idRegTest=3208_

at Cub Scouts, during your lunchtime at work, or while you're waiting for a haircut.)

- Are there days when I will have at least one hour to devote to focused exam prep? (Examples: time on the commuter train, after the kids go to bed, before anyone else wakes up in the morning).

If you can carve out five one-hour blocks of uninterrupted time per week, there's a high likelihood that you'll be able to adequately prepare before the day of the exam.

Action steps: Take that online quiz related to time management. Write your answers to the bullet-point questions above.

Prioritize Tasks and Estimate Your Time

People often ask me how much time they need to allot for exam prep. This concern is often magnified in those who have failed the exam in the past year. There is no simple answer. Everyone has different learning gaps, and everyone absorbs information at a different speed. It's important, though, to distinguish between the amount of *information* you need to master, and the amount of *time* it takes to master that information. The former can be measured by the number of topics or questions; the latter is measured in number of hours.

Start by figuring the amount of information you need to master. First—if you've taken the IBLCE exam before—look at the score report you received from IBLCE, particularly the per-section scores. Then, consider all the topics and subtopics on the IBLCE Detailed Content Outline. Next, see if you can generate some sub-subtopics. (For example, the outline mentions nipple variations as a subtopic. How many nipple variations can you think of that might be included?)

Prioritize Content Topics and Chronological Areas

If there are any topics that you feel you have completely mastered, don't plan to spend another minute learning about them! Instead, identify the topics and subtopics about which you feel **least** confident. An "easy-peasy" topic for one exam candidate might be a "difficult" topic for another. Consider both the disciplines and the chronological areas.

Over the years that I've been helping people to pass the IBLCE exam, I've identified a few patterns that stand out:

- Dietitians, La Leche League leaders, childbirth educators, and others who focus on support and counseling rarely score high on the pharmacology questions.
- Nurses tend to stumble more often on subtopics related to counseling, nutrition and biochemistry.
- Many candidates have trouble with content related to public health and infant development.
- Everyone--and I mean everyone!--struggles mightily with the research component of the exam. Historically, IBLCE exam candidates score the *lowest* in this area.
- Those who work with newborns tend to do better with test items involving babies from birth to about 1 month of age than they do with test items pertaining to older babies.
- Those who have not worked in a hospital tend to lose points on items about newborns, birth practices, and hospital-based issues.
- Those who have worked primarily with healthy mother-baby pairs lose points when facing items about situations in which the mother or the baby has a health problem (including prematurity.)

Estimate the Time You'll Need

It's vitally important to estimate the number of hours you'll need for each topic. I can't tell you exactly how many hours you, or anyone else, will need--again, it depends on your learning gap and how fast you absorb information. It can be hard to figure this out, and I suspect that most people underestimate, initially. Remember: you'll be taking a comprehensive exam so you'll need a comprehensive approach to prepare for it!

Use the list of topics and subtopics that you created. Next to each subtopic, write how many hours you think you need in order to adequately prepare yourself for the IBLC exam. Allow yourself *at least* two hours for each subtopic. Assume you will need more--sometimes much more--for the topics which are likely to be more challenging for you.

Action Steps: Download the Detailed Content Outline. Highlight the three chronological areas where you feel weakest. Highlight the three disciplines where you feel weakest. Generate a list of subtopics for one of those topics. Assign a number of hours you plan to study in each chronological area, and each discipline.

Set Goals

What goals do you have for yourself? What mini-goals will help you achieve them? Take a moment to list at least three of them. These might be time-bound, such as "Devote six hours a week every week between now and the exam date" or topic-bound, such as, "Complete all course reading assignments pertaining to congenital anomalies." Or, you could use a different taxonomy.

Set mini-goals for yourself, and identify possible obstacles for meeting those goals. If you know what the obstacles might be, you can actively work to eliminate or minimize them. For example, there's a high likelihood that, at some point, your kids are going to have a sick day during time you had planned for study. How will you make up that study time?

Believing that you will indeed reach your goals, plan how and when to celebrate! Celebrate small successes or milestones you achieve throughout your study process. And definitely plan a celebration for when you pass the exam! Assume you will be successful, and recognize the importance of celebrating. Successes spur us on to greater heights, and achieving your goal of IBCLC certification is a fantastic reason for a well-deserved celebration!

Action Steps: Write the three obstacles that are likely to delay the accomplishment of your goals. Make at least a short list of the obstacles that might get in the way of sticking to your schedule. Jot down some ideas for how you can overcome, or at least lessen, those obstacles? Get our free study guide at breastfeedingoutlook.com.

Setting goals, though, isn't enough. A now-famous study by Dr. Gail Matthews at Dominican University showed that people with written goals were 50% more likely to achieve them. You might want to pick up my free 8-week study guide at *breastfeedingoutlook.com* which gives you some structure for setting goals around dates and topics. It's designed with an 8-week timeframe in mind, but you can expand or compress your study effort to meet your needs. If you have an 8-month block, the guide is still a good framework. If you're in a pinch, the plan is flexible enough to be used in a 4-week period, but in general, we recommend no fewer than eight weeks to prepare. Plan at least one milestone you plan to celebrate.

Schedule Study Time

Identifying important dates and deadlines, prioritizing and estimating the time needed, and goal-setting helps to create the structure you need to succeed. Such planning is necessary, but planning is only part of the battle. Next, you must schedule your study time. As time management expert Peter Turla observes, "A plan is WHAT you're going to do; a schedule is WHEN you're going to do it. A to-do item without a time and date is merely a wish."

Scheduling is a cornerstone of structure. By creating a schedule, we know what we need to do and when we need to do it. Here are ten tips to help you schedule (and use!) your study time.

Buy or make a special calendar.

A calendar is essential for managing your time for overall studying, as well as week-to-week or day-to-day studying. Use it to organize your study times, topics, and materials. Review your list of priority topics.

Schedule by working backwards.

Identify the test date, look at today's date, and determine how many weeks remain between now and the exam. List all the topics you need to cover between today and a few days prior to the exam. Then, plug in the topics so that each topic is covered during a particular week. Set aside several hours each week to tackle each topic.

Value your time.

If you truly value your time, you'll develop a schedule and, for the most part, stick to it. Sure, there are times when the schedule needs to be revised, but in general, sticking to the schedule is a way of showing yourself that you value one of your most precious commodities--your time.

Scheduling and using that time is your promise to yourself that you are going to honor something valuable. If you have trouble sticking to your study schedule, consider having an accountability partner.

Use "good" times to study.

In general, studying is most effective when you are rested, when you are alert, and during the time that you've scheduled to study. Try to study at times when you are least likely to have distractions or interruptions. For example, when I'm planning to do some serious studying, I schedule it for long before dawn when I know that there is a low likelihood of having my attention diverted to some issue other than studying. I'm also a "morning person"; if you're not, then you might want to schedule the bulk of your studying at a different time.

Avoid "bad" times to study.

Studying 30 minutes before you try to fall asleep is not a good idea. A friend of mine described it well when he explained, "My body is resting, but my brain is still motoring."

At bedtime, aim to shut off the beta waves associated with learning, and turn on the delta waves that are associated with sleeping. Some people find that studying within 30 minutes of having a substantial meal is not a good idea. This makes sense, since blood that is usually going to your brain is being diverted to the gut for digestion. Plan accordingly.

Use study breaks to your advantage.

Study for about 40-50 minutes at a time, and then take a 10-minute break. Most people do best when they study for many minutes, then take a break for a few minutes. You can even get a Pomodoro app to ding when it's time to take a break and when it's time to return to studying. Studying in larger chunks of time has not been proven effective for retention. Use breaks to refresh and keep going!

Make every minute count.

In other words, study at unscheduled times! Many exam candidates study in short bursts while they are waiting to pick up their children from activities, or while they are waiting for medical or dental appointments. Most use what I call "portable" study materials, such as our *Flashcard App* or audio recordings. Keep in mind that this on-the-spot, quick-study doesn't replace the focused studying that should comprise the majority of your effort. That studying should be done at the time when you're at your best, when you've scheduled it to happen.

Learn about the characteristics of procrastination—and tactics to address it.

I've come to a point where I believe that the urge to procrastinate is part of the human condition. If you've ever put studying on your calendar for a certain date and time, then found yourself organizing your sock drawer or cleaning out your freezer instead, you know what I mean! You then assume that you'll study tomorrow, but, as you've probably noticed, "tomorrow" often brings new distractions that cause you to put off studying until weeks later.

In his book *Solving the Procrastination Puzzle*, Carleton University professor and procrastination researcher Timothy Pychyl explains that the most common reasons for procrastination are that the task is boring, frustrating, ambiguous, unstructured, difficult, or lacking in personal meaning and intrinsic rewards. In my estimation, "unstructured" is the characteristic over which we probably have the most control! (Luckily, Pychyl gives many practical tips for overcoming procrastination.)

Revise your schedule if it isn't working.

Note that the qualifier here is, "if it isn't working." Just putting things off is called procrastination, but revision is a deliberate attempt to make a study schedule that is more effective.

Plan time for taking practice exams.

Everyone--researchers and examinees--agree that practice tests help! However, sometimes, people spend so much time with their nose in a book that they leave themselves no time to take any practice exams.

Plan to take practice tests earlier in your study season. Ideally, practice exams help you figure out your weaknesses and close any learning gaps. Frankly, it does no good to take them the weekend before the exam. If you take them at the last minute and don't do well, it will be a mental downer and you will go into the real exam feeling inadequate for the task. You will have little time to learn the material pertaining to what you haven't yet mastered, but the outcome is still likely to deprive you of some good sleep. Rather than cramming with practice exams at the last minute, research has repeatedly shown that good nutrition and a good night's sleep for several days (or weeks) leading up to the exam are more likely to help you do well on the exam.

I feel compelled to warn against using just recall-only "quiz" questions for your studying. These recall-only questions can be very useful; you can't apply information you can't recall! But you absolutely must schedule time to take a practice exam, which models the test you'll be taking.

To truly mimic the IBLCE exam, a practice test should be designed to occupy about four hours of time, and its questions should be application-based vignettes, since that's what the real exam will have. If you want to take more than one practice exam, or take one practice exam multiple times, allow time for that. (Our practice exams can be taken repeatedly, and allow you to scramble the order of the items.) And, the test items should be little vignettes that are application-oriented, since that's the way the real exam will be.

Action Step: Review the 10 tips listed above. Circle the three tips that are likely to be the most influential in creating your success on the exam.

Gather Materials and Equipment

When you're preparing for a comprehensive exam, getting your materials and equipment together is a little different than when you're preparing for the final exam from a subject-specific course.

To make the best use of your study time, you need to get all of your stuff together before you start. Why so?

Because getting up from your chair to find "something" can be a huge distractor. Instead of returning promptly to your studies, you end up throwing in a load of laundry, or even whipping up a batch of cookies! You risk losing your focus and wasting time. However, gathering what you need can be done in three simple steps.

Step 1: Gather your old course materials.

It may have been awhile since you took the many courses that were required to sit for a comprehensive exam--you may need to set aside time just to locate your course materials! Nevertheless, before you sit down for serious studying, gather your old text books.

Consider whether you want to dig up your old notes. I'm not convinced that exam candidates profit from re-reading their notes. But if you have them and feel sure they will be useful, locate old notebooks, binders, journals, and anything else before you start studying. Looking for them later is just a time-waster.

Step 2: Get your tech and related materials.

You'll for sure want your computer or tablet, and a printer. You will undoubtedly have resources that need to be downloaded, and probably printed. Make a list of those. Be sure your printer has plenty of ink and have a back-up ink cartridge nearby. (Long after midnight when you're standing in your pajamas trying to print something critical, you don't want to discover that you're lacking paper or a new ink cartridge for your printer! Trust me, I've been in that situation!) And, you may want a way to corral and organize the downloaded documents you have printed out with one or more of the office supplies listed below.

Step 3: Gather office supplies.

This means, gather every office supply that might enable you to create the kinds of study experiences that you need. It's not enough to simply re-read your books, articles, and class notes. You'll need to make new notes in various ways. You probably don't need all of these, but if you have all of these handy, you won't need to go looking for them later.

- Pencils with erasers
- Pens
- Colored markers
- Highlighters
- Stapler, small and large paper clips, rubber bands
- Index cards
- Lined paper
- Unlined paper
- Spiral notebook
- 3-hole punch
- 3-hole punched paper
- 3-ring binder
- Newsprint (for large illustrations and/or mind maps)
- Replacement printer cartridges
- Low-sugar snacks
- Water
- Beverage you enjoy: Coffee, tea, lemonade, whatever

If you have everything you need before you start studying, you will be well on your way to avoiding the procrastinating that almost always follows once you become distracted.

Action Steps: I've created a long list for you. Cross out the items that you feel are irrelevant for you or your study needs. Then, schedule a day to locate and/or buy the other items, and do it! You might be surprised how scheduling and completing a simple task like helps you focus and follow through with other tasks!

Create a Good Study Environment

Your study environment can have profound effects on your ability to use your study time wisely. Here are four factors that can affect how efficiently you study:

Sensory stimulation

Anything that you can see, hear, touch, taste, or smell can affect your study time. Research has shown that studying with headphones on tends to decrease memory and information retention. However, background music--if it is familiar--can be helpful. Seeing a beautiful landscape or fresh flowers might be helpful to some, but distracting to others. The aroma of fresh bread baking might be pleasant, but it can also make you hungry and thereby distract you from your studies.

Comfort

Good lighting and comfortable seating is critical. If you've ever experienced eye strain or butt fatigue, you know what I mean! Some people like to study outside, which is great as long as that helps and inspires you, rather than distracts you. Temperature or humidity might bother you. Thunder rumbling in the background can be a distractor. A strong wind that blows papers around is definitely a big distractor!

Room aesthetics

Personally, I can't concentrate in a dark, cluttered, cramped environment. I do much better in a large, brightly lit room. When I first wrote my Lactation Exam Review course, I took a dramatic step: I rented a hotel suite for a few days! I needed that bright, airy feeling (not to mention the freedom from unscheduled distraction) to do my best work. Somehow, the big uncluttered space gives me a big, uncluttered brain. I am not the only person who seeks this.

Give some thought to what sort of room aesthetics help you to concentrate and do your best work, and think about what doesn't.

Variety

Some people find it more stimulating to study in different environments. Some people study at a different coffee shop every day because it makes them feel more stimulated and more motivated. You might not be one of those people. Nonetheless, nearly everyone finds it helpful to get out of the study environment for several minutes; taking a walk can help clear your head so you can come back and study refreshed.

Electronic lures

These days, there are all sorts of electronic gizmos to lure you from your studies--smart phones, email, text messages and more. Learn to use the "do not disturb" option during your study time.

People

However much you may love or enjoy them, people can be a real distraction. If your kids con you into being their playmate, referee, cook or a homework companion, you will be distracted from your studies. If you're in a park or at a coffee shop, you may be distracted by someone who wants to strike up a conversation. Consider some ways to minimize these situations.

Bed

Unless you're that rare person who has developed a habit of productively studying in bed, don't try this. First, you'll probably feel so comfortable that you lose your focus. Just as importantly, though, the bed is for sleeping. Studies have shown that when you do work in your bed, your brain begins to associate the stress of "work" with "bed."

Don't underestimate the influence of your study environment. But understand that what works for one person doesn't necessarily work for another person.

Action Steps: Put a star next to the three factors that you would consider the most important for you to control when selecting your study environment.

· ·

61

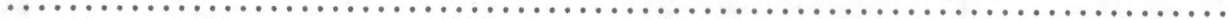

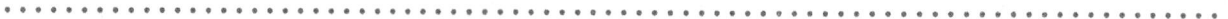

Chapter 10: Plan a Process to Prepare for the Exam

In the last chapter you learned how to plan a structure to support your goal. Certainly, structure is necessary! But a good process is also needed in order to achieve the desired outcome. Before you dive in to the process, plan it carefully. American statesman and founding father Benjamin Franklin advised that "If you fail to plan, you are planning to fail!" In the many years since he uttered those wise words, entire books have been written on the importance of planning.

If your goal is to pass the IBLCE exam, you will need to develop a study plan. In this chapter, I will talk about general methods for studying, specific study techniques, and effective versus ineffective techniques.

Learning is not an event; it is a process. There are several processes by which to learn. Different experts use different words to connote different, similar or the same meaning to explain the processes. I talk about "strategies." The word implies a more strategic, long-term plan to accomplish a learning goal.

Choose Study Strategies

There are five classifications: direct learning, indirect learning, interactive learning, experiential learning, or independent learning. Let's take a look at each of them.

Direct learning methods

Direct learning methods are instructor-directed. In essence, the instructor dispenses information, and the learner passively listens or watches.

By far the most common example of a direct learning method is a lecture, whether delivered in-person or online. This, like other passive means of learning, is highly ineffective for knowledge mastery and retention.

Yet, direct learning methods do offer something critical. The instructor has already identified the information that is relevant to the exam, as well as clinical practice. Whether you've never taken the IBLCE exam before or you've taken it but still feel shaky about how to prepare, including lecture among your study strategies enables you to benefit from her judgment and experience. During the lecture, you can take notes, which you can use for study now and for review later.

However, with rare exception, most learners need more than direct-learning methods. Why? Research in the education field has shown that we retain only a fraction of what we hear. By itself, it's not an effective study strategy.

Indirect learning methods

With indirect methods, the instructor's role changes from one who dispenses information to one who facilitates or supports learning. The instructor arranges the learning environment, provides an opportunity for your involvement, and gives constructive feedback. The learner doesn't just listen passively, but instead takes on a more active learning role by making observations or gaining insights, forming and connecting relevant concepts, and problem-solving.

Examples include guided discussion of case studies, journal clubs, and group discussion.

Indirect learning methods can be highly effective methods for learning new information and/or reviewing previously-mastered information. However, to be effective, this method requires a skilled instructor; most learners are unable to use indirect learning methods without expert guidance.

Interactive methods

Interactive methods involve the learner in their own learning. Common examples of interactive methods used in the classroom include role-playing, discussion, or debates. However, interactive methods can also be used outside of the classroom; a common example is participating in a weekly study group, or completing group projects.

Because learners use their whole body--talking, listening, doing and often, moving--interactive methods are highly effective. However, interactive methods usually don't work at all without a pre-determined structure. Hence, a study group that meets outside of the classroom won't be effective if it has a "let's get together sometime and study this stuff" approach.

Experiential methods

Experiential methods put the learner in the field. Taking a field trip to a museum, conducting an experiment in a lab, or playing a relevant game are all excellent examples of experiential learning methods.

The role of the learner may be to observe (e.g., viewing art in the museum) or to actively participate (e.g., conducting an experiment in the lab). In the field of healthcare, actively delivering client care is an excellent example of an experiential learning method.

To gain the most from your clinical experience, develop a clearly-defined structure for your learning, keeping in mind all of the topics on the ***IBLCE's Detailed Outline***.

Independent methods

Independent methods are those in which the learner works without an instructor or peers. Examples include reports, essays, homework, or similar activities. In my estimation, few individuals learn well with these methods unless an instructor has provided **substantial** structure. One exception, however, is the learning journal.

A learning journal enables you to reflect on your learning process. Studies show that use of a learning journal supports better learning.

I located at least ten studies showing the benefits of using a learning journal. These included greater assimilation and integration of new information, better long-term retention of course concepts, better test and exam grades, and continuous feedback about one's own learning. To get started, take a look at the Penzu template or consider an app.

Knowing that you must get ready for a comprehensive exam, you may be tempted to dive right in and begin reading or watching everything you can get your hands on related to breastfeeding. But that's unlikely to give you a solid understanding of the many subjects you need to know for the IBLCE exam. I encourage you instead to think about what approaches you can use to study, and which means will help you reach your ultimate goal of passing the IBLCE exam.

Action Steps: Venture out a little! Instead of using the same strategies you've been using, jot down three strategies that you've never tried before, and commit to trying them. (If you hate the ones you picked, you can switch to something different, but at least try!)

Choose Study Techniques

Once you've chosen your study strategies, it's time to think about techniques (also called methods). These are the observable actions within one of those strategies. For example, if you join a study group, that's an interactive (also called "cooperative") learning strategy, but at any given time, the study group may use one or more learning techniques, such as role-play or problem-solving. For our purposes, I'd like to talk about learning techniques.

Techniques used by most students

Dunlosky and colleagues (2013) published an enormously helpful study about the effectiveness of learning techniques. First, they listed commonly-used study techniques:

- Highlighting/underlining (marking while reading)
- Re-reading (reading the text again, after having done it previously)
- Elaborative interrogation (explaining a fact)
- Self-explanation (steps in problem-solving)
- Summarization (writing summaries)
- Keyword mnemonic (association of keywords and mental imagery)
- Imagery for text (attempting a "photographic" memory)
- Practice testing (taking practice exams)
- Distributed practice (learning small chunks at one time)
- Interleaved practice (mixing different problems)

Action Steps: Using the 10 techniques that Dunlosky and colleagues studied, circle the three that you've used most frequently in the past.

The study results should be of interest to those who are preparing for a comprehensive exam. I've helped literally thousands of people to prepare for the IBLCE exam; **nearly all who talk with me say they rely almost entirely on highlighting while reading,** or re-reading material they have previously read.

Least effective techniques

Highlighting and re-reading were both found to have very low utility. Of highlighting, the authors said that it "does little to boost performance...it may actually hurt performance on higher-level tasks that require inference-making."

Re-reading was also rated as having very low utility. The authors pointed out that a major reason for ranking it as having low utility was that it was not as effective as other techniques. (It was not apparent if the authors were referring to re-reading only the textbook, or if re-reading included the re-reading of class notes.) Re-reading appeared to be somewhat useful for recall-based test items, whereas "the benefit for comprehension is less clear." Again, since the IBLCE exam requires the candidate to have at least comprehension--and usually application--relying on re-reading as a major or only learning technique is inadvisable.

Moderately effective techniques

Dunlosky and colleagues gave an overall rating of "moderate" to the other six strategies. This was, in part, because the techniques were effective with some tasks, some groups (older or younger) or various other circumstances, but they did not have high utility across the board. Although they gave a clear rationale for why they picked the 10 techniques they studied, they did say that many other techniques were simply not discussed in the study.

So we see two techniques that had low utility, and six that had moderate utility (depending on the circumstances). What were the other two? Ah, yes! Practice exams, and distributed practice!

Most effective techniques

This extensive, well-designed study showed that practice exams and distributed practice ranked as being the most effective study techniques. To quote their study, "Practice testing and distributed practice received high utility assessments because they benefit learners of different ages and abilities, and have been shown to boost students' performance across many criterion tasks and even in educational contexts."

Here's the bottom line: If you're highlighting and re-reading, you are using the LEAST effective study strategies. Instead, you should be using practice tests, and some form of distributed practice! (One example of distributed practice is flash cards, which has been a huge favorite among my course participants for over a decade.) You should also consider using some of the moderately effective techniques.

Predict the LIKELY Exam Questions

It's often helpful to try and predict what questions the IBLCE could be likely to ask. Start with a topic you know well, and then try to make progressively more difficult questions to go along with the topic. For example, the IBLCE Content Outline lists "Nipple structure and variations" as an exam topic. What do you think they might ask about the nipple structure and variations?

Simple Recall Questions

Simple recall involves retrieving previously-learned information. Here are some ideas that could be worked into a multiple-choice, simple-recall test item:

- What's the definition of a nipple? What characteristics would one expect to find on a normal nipple?
- Given a photo, can you identify a normal nipple on a fetus, a newborn, an infant, a child, an adolescent, a non-lactating mother, a lactating mother?
- Given a drawing, would you be able to label all six layers of skin tissue on a normal nipple?
- Can you give a list of characteristics of a normal nipple? (Size, shape, color, placement in relation to the surface of the skin, etc.)

Comprehension Questions

Comprehension is about discovering the meaning of information. Here are some ideas that could be worked into a multiple-choice test item that deal with discovering information

- What do you think IBLCE means by a "variation" of normal?
- What might be an example of a nipple variation that is simply part of the woman's basic anatomy?
- What might be an example of a nipple variation that has been acquired through surgery, injury, or some other means?
- Given a photo, could you classify a nipple as normal, abnormal, or a variant of normal?

- Could you give a list of possible nipple variations?
- Could you describe variations that the woman was born with (such as an inverted nipple) versus a nipple variation that anyone might acquire (perhaps due to surgery, or something else) versus something that is a variation that would occur in a lactating mother, but not a non-lactating mother?
- Could you distinguish one type of congenital nipple variation from another?
- Could you locate where the nipple is in relation to the body of the breast, in relation to the nerves that innervate the sensation and function of the nipple, or where it is in relation to the vessels that supply it with blood?
- Could you explain what might have caused a nipple to become cracked or bleeding?
- Could you select technology to help correct some nipple problem?
- Could you name the number of sprays that would likely come out of the nipple?
- What type of infection is likely to be on the nipple, but unlikely to be in other locations unless it is also on the nipple?
- What sorts of devices might be used to correct nipple variations or abnormalities?

Application Questions

Application is using previously-learned information in new ways. Here are some ideas that could be worked into a multiple-choice exam item:
- Could you implement a strategy to help a woman who had some type of nipple variation to effectively latch her baby on?
- From a legal/ethical standpoint, how would you help a mother with nipple blebs?
- How might having a pierced nipple alter the overall plan of care for the mother?
- What points would you need to make in teaching a woman who has been given topical medication for her nipples?
- How would you use one or more devices to help a mother with a nipple variation?
- Using what you have learned, how would you solve....
- What approach would you use to ...
- If a mother objected to using animal products, what other product(s) might be helpful for her sore, cracked nipples?

- If a mother has been taking antibiotics, can you predict what organism(s) or condition is likely to result in/on the mother's nipples?
- If a mother reported having sore nipples, what questions would you use in an interview to help the mother and/or physician to resolve the problem?
- How would you use what you have learned to develop a plan of care related to the mother's ability to breastfeed with a specific nipple variation?

Analysis Questions

Analysis is a break-down of component parts to identify motives or causes, make inferences, determine relationships, or draw conclusions. Analysis isn't easy, but you should be prepared for at least a few questions that require analysis. Here are some ideas:

- Can you list the layers of nipple skin and relate them to location of nerves and therefore to perception of pain and pleasure in the nipples? Notice that "list" is only part of what you'd need to do; you'd need to relate this list to a clinical implication.
- What is the relationship between specific breaks in nipple skin (e.g., blisters, ulcers, cracks) and specific problems with infant latch?
- Given a photo showing the variation, can you distinguish between nipples that will affect breastfeeding outcomes, and those that will not?
- Can you cite at least five examples of inaccurate advice that women are commonly given about how to prevent or solve issues of sore nipples during pregnancy or lactation?
- Evaluation (Making judgments on the basis of given criteria)

Synthesis Questions

Synthesis is about applying prior knowledge and skills to produce something new. This is almost always going to be along the lines of creating a plan of care with some unusual circumstances. Let's say that the question asks about which hold you would be LEAST likely to suggest for a nursing couplet. In the stem, it says that the mother suffers from carpal tunnel syndrome. In that case, you must synthesize your knowledge of positioning and latch with your understanding of carpal tunnel, and how it would affect the mother's ability to use a cross-cradle hold.

Action Steps: Think about the questions posed for application-level questions. What sorts of questions would be difficult for you to face on the exam?

Use Techniques for Focus and Follow-Through

Anyone who has ever set a goal for anything--losing weight, paying off a credit card, or preparing for a comprehensive exam--knows that oftentimes, as the saying goes "the spirit is willing, but the flesh is weak." There are several tips that can help us to focus, and follow through.

Develop good habits, routine, or rituals. As Benjamin Franklin said, "Your net worth to the world is usually determined by what remains after your bad habits are subtracted from your good ones." If you feel your net worth to your exam success is because of your bad study habits, you can fix that! Develop more good study habits, get rid of some bad study habits, or do both!

Find "carrots and sticks" to motivate you.

In the common lingo, "carrots" are our rewards, they are the motivators that keep us moving towards our goal. "Sticks" are the punishments, they help keep us from slacking off since we don't want to suffer them.

These days, neither carrots nor sticks need to be tangible. They can be online! Check out *StickK.com*. You can commit on the web site to do or not do a particular activity. For example, you might say you will do exercise four times this week, or complete three hours of studying for the IBLCE exam; you might say you will not smoke cigarettes this week. You sign a legally-binding online contract, and you decide what stakes you want to put on the line. If you fail to meet your goal, you pay the stakes. You can also pick people to receive emails that update them on your progress We know that research has shown that having an accountability partner can help keep you on track when working towards a goal. StickK.com is a way of being your own accountability partner. Or, use it with a real partner. You can both set your goals, receive emailed updates about your mutual progress, and identify each other as the party to receive the reward if a goal is unmet.

Get rid of digital distractions. If you are tempted to surf the web, you can get a website blocker, such as SelfRestraint (PC) or Self-Control (Mac). If your software (like your email!) is getting in your way, try a software blocker, such as Concentrate or Think.

Use time-trackers to track the time you spend studying.

RescueTime for the PC or Mac is a web-based cross-platform. The dressed-down version is free, or you can buy a subscription for the upgrade. This popular program helps you make sure you keep your study schedule. If you don't like a web-based app, consider Toggl, also available in a basic free version or as a monthly subscription. There are other alternatives, too, but it appears that these are the most established and most popular time-trackers.

Use productivity-enhancing tools.

I've tried more than a dozen apps that promise to enhance productivity, and I prefer ones that are streamlined and easy to use. Otherwise, I find myself spending more time tinkering than doing my work. With so many apps available, I would suggest that you download one that is free. Popular apps include Wunderlust, ChecklistPro Lite, Reminders, To-Do, Any DO (my personal favorite, since it is easy to use and allows me to speak my entries rather than type them.)

Empower yourself by seeing your progress.

Several apps give you the ability to give yourself credit for something you do repeatedly. Let's say that your goal is to study one hour on Monday, Tuesday, Thursday, and Friday each week, beginning at 5:30 AM. You can set up your app to help you develop that habit. I have used both Habits and Streaks, but if those two don't appeal to you, there are plenty of others.

Action Steps: Write down at least two techniques you can use to help yourself get focused.

Chapter 11: Master Test-Taking Strategies

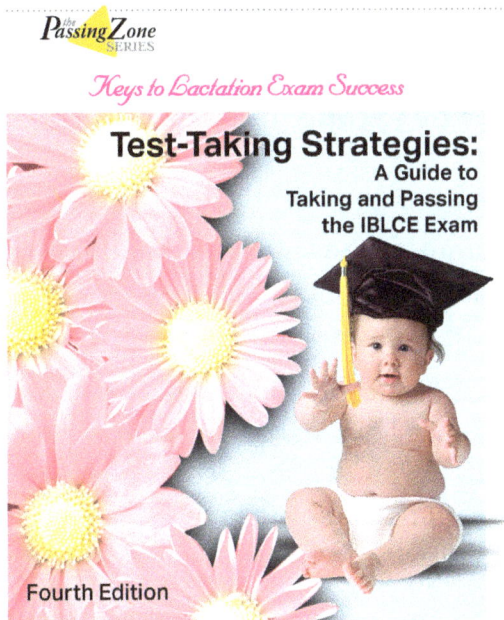

PassingZone SERIES

Keys to Lactation Exam Success

Test-Taking Strategies:
A Guide to Taking and Passing the IBLCE Exam

Fourth Edition

by Marie Biancuzzo RN MS IBCLC

Studying information on breastfeeding and lactation, and having clinical experience will play a big role in your success on the Exam. However, you'll also need to plan to spend some time brushing up on a non-clinical skill: test-taking. As a first step, review the anatomy of a test item and the headsets around test-taking in Unit 1.

To some extent, your results will be affected by how good you are at test-taking. The following strategies will help you prepare for the IBLCE exam--or, really, any exam.

Know what to do when you know the answer.

Pay attention to any qualifier in the stem or the options. Eliminate any options that you know are incorrect. Here are some tips:

Answer the easy items first. This boosts your morale, and because you can do it quickly, it will give you more time to deal with the items about which you are less confident.

Note the qualifiers. Here are some qualifiers that typically occur in the stem: most, least, except, first, last, only, primarily, and best. There are probably others, but these are the most likely ones. Stick with your first answer! In general, the first answer you write down is usually the correct one. So, follow your gut; you are probably right. Do not second-guess yourself. Do not change your answer unless you are absolutely certain that you made a mistake.

Respond even when you feel a little uncertain.

If you're like me, there are plenty of test situations that make you feel uncertain so bolster your powers of recall. Visualizing real-life situations, using etymology (prefixes, suffixes and roots) are ways to help you along. Finally, knock off at least one or preferably two of the distractors! Remember, they are just distractors!

Guess, when you are completely stumped!

When you are completely stumped, you should guess! Now, I mean you should guess when you are completely, totally, 101% stumped. There is no penalty for guessing, so just do it!

My popular book, *Test-Taking Strategies* includes these tips, and many more. I originally wrote the book because I spent so much time after my Lactation Exam Review helping people develop some test-taking savvy. If you are intimidated by the idea of taking an exam, or if it's been a while since you have, this book may be just the thing for you!

Action Steps: Write down the FIRST thing you want to do to improve your test-taking skills!

Chapter 12: Consider Special Resources

Some of the following resources have been mentioned earlier in this book, but they bear calling-out for special mention. What might work well for one person won't necessarily work well for another, but read on to consider some strategies that may help ensure you succeed in preparing for the IBLCE exam, including: a learning journal, an accountability partner, a study group, and professional help.

Learning Journal

Typically, a learning journal is a collection of notes, observations, helpful resources, conversations with mentors, thoughts, insights, feelings, and more. The purpose of the journal is to provide a go-to place for information that will help you to be more insightful about your learning experience, from both cognitive and affective standpoints. The journal can be an excellent tool to help you identify your strengths and weaknesses related to exam preparation. Research has repeatedly shown the value of journaling for academic or other reasons.

When I was in nursing school, some course instructors required us to keep a journal about our learning experience throughout the semester. At first, I thought it was just a time-waster. Eventually, though, I began to see the usefulness of recording not only what I had learned, but what I wanted to learn, how I was most likely to learn best, and how I felt about the learning that had or hadn't take place.

I still keep a learning journal, although now its focus is more about the insights I have gained through the journal articles I have collected and read. I started with spiral notebooks and handwritten notes. Later, I began typing my thoughts, printing them, and arranging them in 3-ring notebooks under specific subjects. Now, I use Evernote for making notes and attaching resources. You might like to use an online resource like Penzu, although there's nothing wrong with paper and pencil if you prefer to go "old school"!

Action Steps: Take a piece of paper, and fold it in half, length-wise. On one side, write what you consider the pros of keeping a learning journal. On the other side, write what you consider the cons. There are no right or wrong answers; everyone has a different perception!

Accountability Partner

You want to do it. You really do. But no matter how often you tell yourself you're going to take--and rock--the next step of your IBCLC journey, you just don't do it. There's another voice inside your head telling you, just as often, that you can't. Or that you won't. Or that you don't need to. Or that it is too hard. The list of internal objections seems almost endless. What can you do?

Often, the difference comes when you take the intentions you've thought and speak them, especially to another person. Telling someone what you are going to do can often be a powerful step in cementing your intentions. But who you tell--and what you and they do afterwards--can make the difference between your success and your failure. That's why I recommend an accountability partner, someone who will listen to your goals, act as a sounding board, and hold you accountable in an agreed-upon way if you fail to meet them. This might be your spouse or a friend, but it could be a mentor, a relative, a colleague, or a paid business coach.

Many people find an accountability partner helpful in meeting personal goals--Weight Watchers and Jenny Craig are built on the idea of accountability, and many "gym buddies" or "marathon buddies" find the agreement to exercise together at a scheduled time to be a strong enough incentive to keep them on track. Some breastfeeding mothers find this "buddy system" helpful in the first days or weeks with their new baby. It's become a popular tool for new start-ups and entrepreneurs, too.

How can we apply that to this professional goal? Well, the idea is similar. You communicate with your accountability partner on a routine basis to review your overall goal, set and report on short-term objectives, and discuss any problems that arise.

The IBCLC-path accountability partner can help you think about strategies to prepare--flash cards for vocabulary training perhaps, a cram course if you're stuck at the planning and organization phase, or something else--and keep you honest about taking the steps you need to succeed. It may be helpful to you to set consequences for steps along the way. Some people pay their accountability partner money if they fall short of their goals; others use positive incentives like a celebration or "pay off" if they achieve their goal. Consider what might work for you.

Action Steps: Take a piece of paper, and fold it in half, lengthwise. On one side, write what you consider the pros of having an accountability partner. On the other side, write what you consider the cons. There are no right or wrong answers; everyone has a different perception!

Study Group

Research shows that being part of a study group can be more effective than simply studying alone at one's desk. I don't dispute that. Unquestionably, being actively involved in the learning process improves one's ability to learn.

What I seriously question is, will this work for all learners in all study groups? To me, that answer depends on three factors: First, is the learner an introvert or an extrovert? Second, could the learner carry out a different type of active learning strategy—alone or with others? Finally, is it possible that study groups are effective only if they meet certain criteria?

Extroverts tend to do better with study groups than introverts. By definition, extroverts get their energy from other people, and a study group can help them make the most of energy, ideas, and insights of others. Introverts might find the extra stimulation to be counterproductive.

Other active learning strategies might be more effective for some learners. I've mentioned several in this publication, e.g., flash cards, creating written summaries, and more.

If you plan to join a study group, it's good to know what criteria may indicate successfulness. Effective study groups tend to share several critical characteristics:

- well-articulated goal
- clearly-stated "ground" rules for who will do what, when, and how. This includes ground rules for kicking a slacker out of the group, if needed
- an effective, organized leader who can foster good group dynamics, and keep the discussions from veering onto tangents or socializing

- fewer than five high-achievers who are well-prepared each week for their presentation; these don't have to be friends
- a consistent schedule for meeting each week for an agreed upon amount of time, not to exceed two hours or so in length, which is moderated by a timekeeper
- a meeting place that is free of distractions. This includes, but is not limited to, socializing.
- a structure for each meeting, including the identification of unanswered questions at the end of the session and a plan for how to structure the next week's session
- cooperation and agreement from members on salient topics, questions, and problems, as well as offering of study tips and helping to support and motivate other group members

Unless you can join (or start) a study group with these criteria, you are likely better off finding other ways to study. All too often, study groups become free-flowing, unstructured sessions that have no aims, and accomplish little.

If you have already found yourself a study group that does not meet *all* of these criteria, muster the strength to simply remove yourself from the group. It may feel awkward but remember, you are preparing for a high-stakes, career-critical exam. Don't waste your time just because you are afraid of what the group members might think. Remind yourself, the goal here is to pass the exam on the very next try.

Action Steps: Take a piece of paper, and fold it in half, length-wise. On one side, write what you consider the pros of joining a study group. On the other side, write what you consider the cons. There are no right or wrong answers; everyone has a different perception!

Professional Help

It may seem ironic: The same people who are seeking a credential to provide professional help for others frequently don't seek professional help for their own needs. They think they can go it alone. Some can but many others end up failing the exam. Even if they fail, they might not look for professional help. All too often, they buy an additional book or two, talk to a few colleagues, but still try to go it alone.

Why don't people seek professional help? In my experience, these are the most common reasons:

- **Fear and shame**. After failing the exam, it's normal to feel fear or shame, and not want anyone to know what's happened.
- **Feelings of weakness**. This is a bit different than fear and shame. Whereas fear and shame are more about exposure, this is more about feeling a lack of control over the outcome.
- **Denial**. Feelings of denial can lead the exam-taker to believe their experience was a one-time shortcoming that won't happen again.
- **Misperceptions**. Some people don't know how professional help can make a difference, while others wonder if such courses are little more than money-making schemes.
- **Family or work scheduling**. Getting professional help might mean committing to a specific time or date, which you may write off as too difficult before you investigate all your options.
- **Financial barriers**. Paying for the IBLCE exam is itself a pricey endeavor so you might initially cringe at adding exam prep costs. But if you don't get professional help and try to go it alone, you might fail altogether.
- **Hopelessness**. Some test-takers feel that they are so bad off that nothing can help them. When they accept professional help, they often find out that's not the case. One woman who hesitantly accepted my help went on to increase her IBLCE exam score by 15 points! That's a lot!

Certainly, a successful candidate must have some personal competencies and characteristics to succeed: discipline, motivation, and time management skills all figure into the success equation. But if you've taken and failed the exam, it may be time to reach out for experienced help. And why not?

We all seek help from others on a regular basis. If your home needs to be re-wired, you look for a professional electrician. If your car's transmission fails, you hire a professional auto mechanic. If a filling falls out of your molar, you hire a professional dentist to replace it. If you are accused of a crime, you hire a professional attorney. If you don't seem to have enough milk for you baby, you hire a...oh wait. You *would* hire a professional lactation consultant, right?

There is nothing wrong with seeking professional help. All of us do it in many other contexts every day of the week. We expect the mothers and babies to contact us when they need breastfeeding help. It makes sense to feel just as comfortable seeking help for exam prep when it's needed. In many cases, getting professional help can be the difference between an undesired outcome, and a desired outcome.

Chapter 13: Celebrate a Successful Outcome!

Author Robert Black notes that "gambling is a fascinating sport. When you are winning, you are like a human hurricane, nothing can stand in your way." Even if you don't gamble, you can appreciate the truth of this statement. If you have ever been aware of your winning streak at anything--card games, basketball games, or the game of life--you will indeed feel like a human hurricane. Awareness, though, is key. That's why celebrating small successes is so critical. In celebrating small successes, you begin to develop focus and gather momentum.

It's imperative to keep your eye on the "big goal." But it's also important to have micro-celebrations along the way.

You might ask, what constitutes a celebration? When and how should we celebrate? Leadership expert Kevin Eikenberry gives suggestions for *what and when* to celebrate (he calls these "results" components) as well as *how* to celebrate (what he calls "process" components).

Nearly all of Eikenberry's suggestions relate to group celebrations in a business environment, so I have created questions that are more relevant to the process of preparing for and taking a career-critical exam.

- What milestones deserve a celebration? If you have set up your study structure, you'll have plenty of milestones to pick from, including completing tasks, meeting with an accountability partner, achieving a certain score on a practice exam, or any other number of smaller milestones that are helping you to achieve your ultimate goal.
- Who can help you celebrate? Maybe your kids, or your colleagues, or your social media contacts. How about sharing your progress on Facebook or Twitter?
- Who should you thank? Few of us succeed without help from at least one other person. Be sure to call or drop an email or a note to anyone who has helped you to get this far. Messages of gratitude benefit both the recipient and the sender.

- What keeps the celebration in perspective? While you might have rightfully planned a big reward for yourself when you achieve your big goal, don't overdo it for the milestones.
- What, exactly is a celebration? Honestly, it includes anything that acknowledges your sense of accomplishment. It might be as simple as a fist-pump by yourself or a high-five with someone else. It could be a simple pleasure that you enjoy but don't always allow yourself to have: a long walk, a decadent dessert, or a day wandering around a museum. If your budget is bigger, you could plan anything that you would consider a treat: a mani/pedi, a full day at the spa, a weekend at the beach, or a designer handbag. The key here is reflection and recognition. If you don't take the time to recognize your efforts, you will not realize how far you have come, and you run the risk of losing both focus and momentum.

A popular meme, often incorrectly attributed to author C.S. Lewis, observes: "Isn't it funny how day by day nothing changes, but when you look back everything is different?" When we celebrate, we are more likely to shift our perspective on the day-to-day events. Sure, after passing the exam, you can look back and everything will look different. But arranging a small celebration helps you to recognize progress and often gives a boost that will keep you going.

Chapter 14: Summary

To recap, if you have taken the IBLCE exam unsuccessfully, consider these 15 words today:

1. Pause

It was a big blow. Pause. You didn't take the IBLCE exam hoping to fail, and if that's happened, you probably feel like you have been sucker-punched. You may have put a lot of time and energy into passing. You may feel like you've been preparing for this exam for your whole life, and failing is a big blow.

Give yourself a week or two before you decide whether you're going to try again. But if you're serious about becoming an IBCLC, make sure that's a brief pause, not a prolonged stall. There's a difference. You'll need to get up again fairly soon, dust yourself off, and figure out your new approach.

2. Protect

Protect yourself from the people who offer pity. Protect yourself from people who want to blame the IBLCE, the exam proctor, the temperature of the room, or other factors out of your control. Protect yourself from people who start making up excuses for you, or offer their own war stories of how their grandmother died the night before the exam, or their bifocals were inadequate for seeing the pictures.

People who offer pity can't control one thing in future exams, and neither can you. Blame, excuses, and denial won't get the job done. If you want to pass, allow yourself to take full responsibility for your own actions and omissions.

3. Probe

Look at that analysis sheet which the IBLCE sent to you. Note areas where you were strong, and areas where you were weak.

If you don't understand what those categories mean, call my office at 703-787-9894. We're a full-service educational and consulting company. Our staff is specially trained to know those categories inside and out, and we're happy to take time to help you figure them out, too. Without probing the depths of that analysis sheet, you can't get to the next step, which is pinpointing what you can fix about your exam prep.

4. Pinpoint

Pinpoint your weaknesses. Notice I said "weaknesses." Stop kidding yourself by calling a failing score a "challenge." See the situation as it is; no better than it is and no worse than it is. Because of your strengths, you picked some right answers, and because of your weaknesses you picked some wrong answers. Once you pinpoint your weaknesses, *then* you have a challenge: to transform them into strengths.

So what are you trying to pinpoint? Sure, when you probe the analysis of your last exam results, you will have some clues about the content the exam covered. But there are a whole bunch of other factors--including your test-taking skills and anxiety level--that can impact your score. Pinpointing is important.

5. Pack

That's right: Pack your bags. Request days off from work, line up childcare, and pack what you will need to attend an in-person exam prep course.

I distinctly recall a woman who traveled halfway around the world to come to my course. It seemed like an arduous undertaking for the purpose of taking a course! I wasn't sure that I would do it myself, but her story was compelling.

She had completed an online course I'd never heard of, taken the IBLCE exam, and failed. She then repeated the do-it-yourself course, and she failed the IBLCE exam a second time. She explained that a face-to-face course offered her the advantages she needed to pass. Although none of my other exam prep students have traveled as far, many others have identified the same advantages.

Being free from the kids, the dog, the job, and similar real-life distractions allows you to hunker down. Furthermore, an in-person instructor can read your non-verbal cues and offer help on the spot, at the break, or after class. An online course can't do that!

Online courses can be good, but if a do-it-yourself endeavor didn't help you to achieve a passing score last time, you'll want to try an approach with more hands-on help when you retake. Pack your bags, and give yourself a chance to become completely immersed in your learning experience.

6. Participate

Participate in something. Anything. But participate. Participate in a course, participate in a study group, do some learning exercises, buzz through some flash cards. Notice a kid in the elevator, guess his age, and then ask the mother if you're right. Anything that involves active learning increases your chances of passing the next exam.

Look at how much active learning you did when you prepared for your last IBLCE exam. Did you do an all online course? Were you taught mostly through lectures and video? That means you earned the necessary credits. That means knowledge was dispensed to you. That doesn't mean you learned. Don't confuse the completion of credits, time, and teaching with learning. Unless you learn, you won't pass the IBLCE exam.

Over the years, educational research has shown that people retain only about 10% of what they read or hear and only about 30% of what they see on videos. Admittedly, the numbers vary some from study to study, but education experts agree that passive learning through lectures and videos is not as effective as active learning. If you value evidence-based strategies for optimal healthcare outcomes, you should value evidence-based strategies for educational outcomes.

Think about what you're doing, or have done: Are you going to take the same approach again? Doing more of the same strategy is likely to have exactly the same outcome as before, not catapult you into exam success.

7. Plan

Plan your exam prep structure. If you don't have a multi-month structure for yourself, you are writing your ticket to failure. You need to devise a clear plan that maps out when and what you're going to study. Otherwise, you'll find yourself a month away from the exam, you'll study just the topics you enjoy, and you won't learn the stuff you really need to learn in order to pass the exam.

Last-minute cramming is ineffective in helping you get to your goal, which is passing! Along with that, you should plan to succeed. As the old saying goes, **if you fail to plan, you are planning to fail.**

8. Prepare

Prepare, prepare, prepare. Legendary basketball coach Bobby Knight gave some advice that's good on and off the court: "The will to succeed is important, but what's more important is the will to prepare."

If you were going to bake an apple pie, you would get prepared. You would make sure you had the right ingredients: the apples, the sugar, and so forth. And, you would make sure that you actually had the right apples for an apple pie. You would know that some apples--like a Fuji or a Red Delicious--are great for eating but don't work well as a pie filling. You would have the basic skills for how to peel the apples, and how to measure the sugar. You might not be highly skilled in rolling out a tender, flaky crust, but you could ask for a little help from someone who has done it many times and thereby improve your skill. Certainly, you would read the recipe from top to bottom before you began your pie-making endeavor, and then you would re-read each step carefully before moving ahead. You need to be at least this careful when preparing to take a high-stakes exam.

The "recipe" for passing the IBLCE exam is knowing the Detailed Course Outline. Inexplicably, many people ignore this document. If you want to discuss it, give me a call or join me for one of my free webinars. Details are available through the Breastfeeding Outlook web site.

Hands down, the best way to prepare for a comprehensive exam is to take a comprehensive approach. Cobbling together your education with a hodge-podge of courses that interest you or are convenient to get won't give you the comprehensive education you need.

I don't have any hard and fast statistics on this--nor does the IBLCE--but nearly all of the panic-stricken people who tell me they've failed the IBLCE exam report that they did not take a comprehensive course. There are likely two reasons for this.

First, it's human nature to study only the stuff you like to learn. That's great, but the IBLCE exam tests the candidate on a lot of boring and tough content. Left to your own devices, you would have skipped the boring or tough topics, even if you knew they were on the exam.

Second, most people don't have a clear idea of how to get 90 hours' worth of formal, lactation-specific education that will help them to pass the exam. I have taken the IBLCE exam multiple times and I have helped thousands of people to pass the IBLCE exam. **I have spent many more than 90 hours just identifying relevant content** for my comprehensive course; that doesn't count the time I've spent preparing, revising, or delivering that content. I don't see how the person who has never taken the exam could possibly choose content that would cover the breadth of the IBLCE exam. It only makes sense to take a **comprehensive** course to help you pass a **comprehensive** exam!

9. Persist

Basketball Hall of Famer, Rhodes Scholar, and former U.S. Senator Bill Bradley said, "Ambition is the path to success. Persistence is the vehicle you arrive in." I can't name any "successful" person who has become an overnight success. I can name plenty who "failed" but persisted.

- Michael Jordan was cut from his high school basketball team.
- Walt Disney was fired from the *Kansas City Star* because his editor said that Walt "lacked imagination and had no good ideas."
- Elvis Presley was told by the concert hall manager at the Grand Ole Opry that he would be better off going back to truck-driving.
- Colonel Harland Sanders peddled his recipe for fried chicken with 11 secret herbs and spices to more than 1,000 prospects before he found a buyer.

- Lucille Ball was a B-rate actress in 72 movies before she began the *I Love Lucy* series.
- Steven King's first novel was rejected 30 times.
- Conrad Hilton wrote in his autobiography that he was so desperate for cash that he slept in his office chair so that he could rent his own hotel room to a traveler, and by the way, the bellboy put gas in Hilton's car!
- Thomas Edison failed at creating the light bulb more than 10,000 times.

The world would be a poorer place if any of these successful people had given up on their ambitions. And it would be a poorer place if you gave up your ambitions, too! Stay on your path; keep your ambition. But certainly, plan to arrive in that vehicle called persistence.

10. Pretend

That's right. I said pretend. Research in the field of neurolinguistics has repeatedly shown that one of the best ways to connect your subconscious desires to your conscience efforts is by having some sort of outward tangible "thing" that transforms the goal in your head--in this case, passing the test and becoming an IBCLC—to make it more real.

At the risk of having you laugh at me, I'll tell you what I did when I was a senior in nursing school: Nearly every night, I took a pen and wrote, "MBiancuzzo RN"—my name as it would appear on my name badge once I achieved my goal—on a paper, many, many times. Keeping that firmly in sight helped to make my goal a reality. At the time, the research for neurolinguistics didn't exist, but honestly, I do believe that this "pretending" was my ticket to passing the NCLEX on the first try. We become what we think about. The great Mohammed Ali, one of the finest boxers the world has ever known, remarked, "I said I was the greatest, even before I was."

11. Perfect

Perfect your test-taking skills. Remember, I said this isn't all about knowing your content. You also need to psyche yourself into taking the exam, and you need to become a savvy test-taker. Our Test-Taking Strategies book can help.

12. Practice

Practice taking IBLCE-type exams. Don't wait until the last minute; do this well in advance. We have several practice exams available on our Breastfeeding Outlook website.

13. Positive thinking and Prayer

On June 25, 1962, the United States Supreme Court banned prayer in schools. That was more than 50 years ago. But, as my husband likes to say: "As long as there are tests in schools, there will be prayer in schools!" The same could be true of the IBLCE exam!

Even if prayer isn't your cup of tea, you can't go wrong with positive thinking. American author and "positive thinking" guru Norman Vincent Peale wrote more than a dozen books with essentially that message!

Think positive. Stop telling yourself you "can't" do it. Get rid of any negative self-talk. Erase every possible trace of self-doubt. Don't allow yourself to dwell on the fact that you failed before; living in the past won't get you to the future you deserve. True, you failed once. Re-frame that fact. Consider becoming an IBCLC a 2-step process and tell yourself "one down, one to go." Or perhaps you have already failed twice? OK, be sure to remind yourself "third time's the charm!"

14. Perform

Most of us perform best when we are well-rested and relaxed. If you have a structured plan for studying several months in advance, you won't have to do any last-minute cramming. You can go to bed early, get a nutritious breakfast under your belt, stand up straight, take a deep breath, and stroll into the test center with the "I got this" look on your face. You can do this.

15. Pass!

Taking the exam--and passing--may seem like climbing the highest mountain, but it really isn't. You don't need to be a genius, or spend your whole day or whole life glued to your books in order to pass. If that were what it took, I would have undoubtedly failed the IBLCE exam every time I have taken it. I'm not a genius, and I can't let one exam occupy my whole life. Fortunately, I don't need to have that level of genius or intensity and neither do you.

The exam itself takes only a few hours, but those few hours will rarely, if ever, determine whether you pass or fail. The outcome of what you do in those few hours is determined almost entirely by how you think and what you do before you arrive at the testing center. As twentieth-century self-help guru Robert Collier points out: "Success is the sum of small efforts, repeated day in and day out."

About Marie

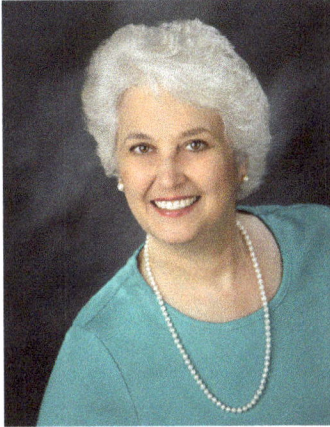

Marie Biancuzzo, Breastfeeding Outlook's Director of Education, has more than 30 years' experience as a clinical nurse specialist in all areas of maternal-child health. A recognized expert in childbearing and breastfeeding, Marie's current work focuses on helping mothers and babies get the care they need—primarily by training health professionals in evidence-based practices.

A founding member of the United States Breastfeeding Committee, and a past president of the Baby-Friendly USA Board of Directors, Marie has been certified by the American Nurses Association as a continuing education specialist, and she was twice chosen to serve on the National Council Licensure Examination (NCLEX) panel of experts that develop the RN licensing exam. She has also been recognized by the International Board of Lactation Consultant Examiners as a long-term provider of continuing education. She has also served on the faculty of three prestigious universities.

Marie has educated thousands of health care professionals through in-person and online seminars and courses. Particularly popular are her Lactation Exam Review, Comprehensive Lactation Course, and Online Lactation Exam Review (podcast format) educational offerings that help health care providers prepare to take the IBLCE exam.

Marie is the author of *Breastfeeding the Newborn: Clinical Strategies for Nurses*, as well as more than 100 articles, a wide variety of independent study modules, and exam prep materials. She is the host of a weekly online radio show, Born to be Breastfed for mothers, lactation professionals, and others. (Currently, more than 70 episodes are available via VoiceAmerica, iTunes or Stitcher.)

Marie is known for the high-quality of her educational programs, as well as her warmth, enthusiasm, and interactive teaching style. You can reach Marie through LinkedIn, Facebook, or at *info@breastfeedingoutlook.com.*

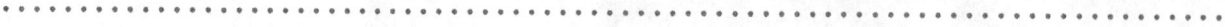

www.ingramcontent.com/pod-product-compliance
Lightning Source LLC
Chambersburg PA
CBHW080001280326
41935CB00013B/1717